Praise for Holly Miller

'Some books rip you apart, even as you are marvelling at how beautifully put together they are. Holly Miller – with her startling metaphors and finely etched portrait of a star-crossed relationship – has created a novel that is unique and breathtaking and painful and broken and perfect . . . just like love'
Jodi Picoult

'What an extraordinary book. It's exquisitely written, incredibly moving and impossible to put down'
Beth O'Leary

'Clever, poignant and very special'
Woman & Home

'A heartrending, beautifully crafted emotional rollercoaster of a read that will stay with you long after the final page'
Mike Gayle

'A love story that will break your heart'
Evening Standard

'A heartbreaking yet heartwarming story'
Prima

'Such a special book. I had a lump in my throat and tears in my eyes to the very last page. I want everyone to read it'
Paige Toon

'An epic love story'
Clare Pooley

'This gorgeous, unusual love story manages to be both heartbreaking and hopeful'
Good Housekeeping

'Utterly moving, this heartfelt read will capture your imagination'
Woman's Own

Holly Miller grew up in Bedfordshire. Since
university she has worked as a marketer,
editor and copywriter. Holly currently
lives in Norfolk with her husband.

Also by Holly Miller

The Sight of You
What Might Have Been
The Spark

Still Falling For You

HOLLY MILLER

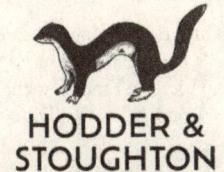

HODDER &
STOUGHTON

First published in Great Britain in 2026 by Hodder & Stoughton Limited
An Hachette UK company

The authorised representative in the EEA is Hachette Ireland, 8 Castlecourt Centre, Dublin 15, D15 XTP3, Ireland (email: info@hbgi.ie)

1

Copyright © Holly Miller 2026

The right of Holly Miller to be identified as the Author
of the Work has been asserted by her in accordance with
the Copyright, Designs and Patents Act 1988.

All rights reserved. No part of this publication may be reproduced,
stored in a retrieval system, or transmitted, in any form or by
any means without the prior written permission of the publisher,
nor be otherwise circulated in any form of binding or cover
other than that in which it is published and without a similar
condition being imposed on the subsequent purchaser.

All characters in this publication are fictitious and any resemblance
to real persons, living or dead, is purely coincidental.

A CIP catalogue record for this title is available from the British Library

Paperback ISBN 978 1 399 70092 4
ebook ISBN 978 1 399 70094 8

Typeset in Plantin Light by Hewer Text UK Ltd, Edinburgh
Printed and bound in Great Britain by Clays Ltd, Elcograf S.p.A.

Hodder & Stoughton policy is to use papers that are natural, renewable
and recyclable products and made from wood grown in sustainable
forests. The logging and manufacturing processes are expected to
conform to the environmental regulations of the country of origin.

Hodder & Stoughton Limited
Carmelite House
50 Victoria Embankment
London EC4Y 0DZ

www.hodder.co.uk

Still Falling For You

SECTION I

1.

Rachel

December 1999

Thirty minutes and seven seconds before the world is due to end, I realise my husband is nowhere to be seen.

'Half an hour left to live, Rach,' my friend Ingrid says solemnly. 'Any final words?'

Millennium eve, and we are in the garden of a country house, deep in the wilds, no neighbours for miles. Which is just as well, because the stereo keeps getting turned up, and everyone should be allowed to choose their own exit music.

'Er, this is a party. Can we do the serious existential shit tomorrow, please?' says my other friend, Polly.

'No, not if we're all dead,' replies Ingrid, reasonably enough, before swigging from the bottle of whisky she's holding.

Polly frowns. She works in IT, has had her fill lately of doomsayers prattling on about nuclear meltdowns and free-falling planes and self-combusting stock markets. Anyway. There are, it seems, more pressing issues at stake.

'Why are you drinking whisky?' she asks Ingrid.

'This is all that's left. We went too early on the champagne.'

'You mean you did,' I say with a smile, turning to scan the garden again for Josh. The rain has cleared from the sky now, and we can finally see the stars.

'Well, it is my last day on earth,' Ingrid says, then fills our empty glasses with enough hard liquor to finish us all off, if Y2K doesn't get to us first.

From the edge of the pool, someone lets off a firework. We watch as it shoots skyward, hanging briefly in the blackness with a whistle, like a bird. Sparks erupt, the air glowing purple and fizzing with gunpowder before an iridescent waterfall descends.

Polly looks down at her whisky-filled champagne flute and shakes her head. 'Oh, this is sad. So very, very sad.'

Ingrid exhales, her breath a spectral twist in the arctic night. 'Right. It's been nice knowing you, but I do have—' she checks her watch '—less than thirty minutes now to line up the best snog of my life.'

'I thought you hated New Year and all its attendant traditions,' I call out as she departs, at which she turns, blows me a kiss, then carries on walking without missing a beat. She is easily the best dressed of everyone here, in black designer taffeta and vertiginous heels, having refused to die with them still in her wardrobe.

Eventually, I spot him. Down by the fence-line, where the edge of the vast garden rolls into a green glimmer of water meadow, Polly's five-year-old son is sitting on my husband's shoulders. Josh is pointing out the stars with a single finger, dancing constellations through the rimy air, showing him the universe. The sight of them together is like a friction burn to my heart.

By my side, Polly nudges me. 'March is your deadline, you know.'

'For what?'

'Having a millennium baby.' She sips her whisky and smiles. 'Might be nice.'

From behind us, her husband Darren chips in. 'Actually, the third millennium doesn't begin until 2001.'

We turn to face him.

He shrugs. 'The AD era starts with year 1.'

Neither of us can be arsed to do the counting backwards.

'Oh, you kept *that* to yourself,' Polly says.

'What, basic arithmetic?'

She snorts. 'So, it's actually this time next year for the apocalypse?'

I watch as Josh begins to walk back towards us, Polly's son still on his shoulders, gripping fistfuls of his hair for balance. 'If you ask Josh, that's probably exactly what he'd say.'

Ten minutes and nineteen seconds until midnight. Josh and I have come inside the house, where he is leading me into the yawning mouth of a long, dark corridor. The silence ticks, and all the lights are off, because the house is so vast, it's not immediately obvious where any of the switches are.

'Josh, this is creepy,' I say, glancing around the galleried walls as we walk, our footsteps echoing against the flagstones. 'All the oil paintings are scowling at us. And there are literal suits of armour.'

'Yeah, but they're guarding something really good. Wait and see.'

'The party's outside.'

'No, the party is very much . . . in here.'

We pause by a heavy wooden door, at which Josh withdraws an enormous wrought-iron key from his pocket.

I lift an eyebrow. 'I think you forgot your kerosene lamp.'

He simply smiles and unlocks the door, heaving it open. It groans and creaks in a way that suggests it hasn't been used since the last time anyone celebrated a millennium.

As I peer past him, a stiff chill ascends. I can see only a flight of steps, swallowed up by a damp-stone darkness, and a banister made of rope. 'You know, if this was a horror film, I'd be saying we deserve everything that's about to happen to us.'

He leans over and flicks on a light. It fizzes and sings, as though the bulb's seconds from blowing. 'Does this help?'

'No. Not in the least.'

'Shall I go first?'

'Do you even need to ask?'

He starts to descend. Nervously, I follow him, hanging on to the rope, just waiting for that door to slam shut and the light to sputter out.

But when we reach the bottom I make a sharp intake of breath.

We are in a cellar with a domed ceiling, every wall lined with rack upon rack of glinting bottles. A tiny cathedral of hedonism, just for us.

I start laughing. 'Oh, my God.'

By my side, Josh beams. 'Ingrid told me where to find the good champagne.'

We nestle down on Josh's jacket, lean back against the chilled stone of the cellar wall.

'We can't take a magnum,' I protest.

'The world's about to end. We can do what we like.'

I suppress a smile. 'I'm surprised you're not out there looting shops.'

'Well, I would be, but . . . I actually had an ulterior motive for bringing you down here,' he says, tugging the cork from the bottle he's picked out.

I smile as it pops. 'Oh, yeah?'

The bulb-light barely stretches to where we are sitting. Josh's face is sliced with shadow, his eyes rich and dark as damp earth. He nods, passes me the champagne. 'Yeah. If there's some sort of biblical explosion up there in the next five minutes, we're essentially in a nuclear bunker, with enough booze to last for another thousand years.'

The bottle's so big, I have to hold it with both hands. I take a swig, the bubbles tart on my tongue, then pass it back to him. 'What about our friends?'

'Ah, screw them. They're going down happy.'

It is silent down here, except for a soft stalactital drip somewhere in the cellar's far corner. Above ground, the music is still pumping.

'You were really sweet with Blake tonight,' I say, picturing him with Polly's son earlier.

He smiles lopsidedly, rubs a hand through his hair. 'Yeah, although he took it too literally when I told him to hold on tight. Virtually scalped me.'

I smile too, then glance at my watch. 'Only two minutes to go. Right. Better say our goodbyes.'

'Can I go first?' Josh sets down the bottle and shuffles round to face me, drawing me in to the low valley of his gaze. 'Well, I should probably just say . . . it's been the privilege of my life to know and love you, Mrs Foster.'

I prod a finger against his ribcage. 'Hey. I don't want be the last thing you ever say to me to be a joke.'

'It's not,' he whispers, then leans forward and kisses me as, above our heads, the clock strikes midnight and the world explodes.

Up there, everywhere could be burning. But down here, right now, we would not know, or care.

2.

Rachel

January 2000

'Has the world ended?' Josh whispers. 'Is everything broken? Burning? Underwater?'

I can't deny that from between the clashing chords of my hangover some notes of relief are breaking through. The world – as far as we know – has remained intact.

Still. No amount of existential solace is going to counteract the effects of that vintage magnum we stole.

'All of the above,' I groan. 'This is my punishment, isn't it, for thieving champagne?'

Josh kisses me, a deep, hotel-room kiss, palms gripping my hips. His skin smells faintly of musk and moss, the fading haze of the night before. I reach beneath the covers, move my hand down, feel him smile.

'Well, technically, *I* thieved,' he says. 'You were just an unwitting accessory.'

'We should punish you, then.'

'Fine by me.' In the lightless bedroom, his fingers skim my underwear. I shut my eyes, feel my heart begin to freewheel as his hand parts my thighs.

Then, a hammering on the door. We jerk away from each other, laughing.

'Hello?' Josh growls, rearranging the quilted bedspread to cover our rapidly heating limbs.

The door swings open. It's Polly's husband, Darren, wearing

a wax jacket and flat cap. This look on him is a touch absurd, given that he's usually to be found scuffing around in trainers and ripped jeans, and is wiry and loose-limbed in a nineties indie band, don't-give-a-shit kind of way.

'Hey,' he says. 'How come you guys got the four-poster?'

Josh tries and fails to smother a laugh. 'What the fuck are you wearing?'

'It's nearly eleven, you pair of wastrels.'

We both just blink at him.

'Time for the pre-lunch Long Walk.'

'You say that like it's a thing,' Josh says.

'It is. Well, today, at least.' Darren strides into the room.

'Go anywhere near those curtains and I won't be responsible for my actions.'

Undeterred, Darren wrenches them open, flooding the room with light. The sky outside is so bright it looks white. 'Come on. Be downstairs in ten minutes.'

'Why are you like this?' Josh says, shading his eyes.

'You can't fester in bed on the first morning of the new millennium.'

'Actually, before you knocked on the door there was very little festering going on.'

'Ten minutes,' he repeats, making a trigger shape with his fingers as he stalks from the room.

'Well, that's obviously not going to happen.' Josh leans into me again as soon as the door clicks shut, but, just as our lips meet, from downstairs someone else calls my name.

'Why are we friends with these people?' I groan, lying back on the mattress.

'They were at the same party as us last night, right?'

'Yeah. And they were drinking last-resort spirits. They should be worse than we are.'

'It's the kids,' he realises. 'All the adults feel like they've been dug up, but the kids have been bouncing off the walls since dawn.'

From downstairs, my name again, more urgent this time. Then, footsteps on the stairs.

'Shit. Darren's sent Polly up.'

'Shit.'

I throw off the bed covers. 'Come on.'

And so, for the second time in twelve hours, we find ourselves hiding from our friends. Only, this time, we're squashed into a cupboard wearing just our underwear, surrounded by fur coats that I hope very much are synthetic.

'This is all very *Chronicles of Narnia*,' Josh says.

'If it's between the witch and a walk, I'll take my chances.'

'Happy New Year,' he whispers, and I stifle a laugh against his bare shoulder as the bedroom door swings open.

To be sure there's no chance of getting frogmarched through Kent, we remain cocooned in the wardrobe. Limbs tangled together, we are cramped but cosy in the gloom, albeit the mothballs are making my nose prickle.

We attempt a kiss, to reignite what we started in bed, but I pull away after a couple of seconds. 'We can't. Not in here.'

Josh smiles. 'Come on. We've never done it inside a cupboard before.'

'It's full of clothes. They might be heirlooms or something. It feels disrespectful.'

'More disrespectful than doing it in their wine cellar? And their bed?'

'I think having sex in someone else's wardrobe would be a new low.'

He laughs, pushes a hand through his dark muddle of hair. 'Yeah, okay. That's fair.'

I feel for his hand, wrap my fingers tightly in his. 'Polly was saying last night we should try for a millennium baby. To sort of . . . mark the moment. You know – being a part of history, and everything.'

'Yeah, I was just waiting to find out if the world's nuclear reactors were still intact.'

'But then Darren reminded us the millennium actually doesn't begin until *next* year.'

He smiles, rests his head against the back of the wardrobe. 'Of course he did.'

'It's a nice idea, though.'

He turns to look at me, his expression gossamer-soft. 'Yeah,' he whispers. 'It's a really nice idea.'

We have always wanted a family of our own. To cultivate something good from the cindered remains of our childhoods. But Josh says – and his eyes say, now – not yet, not yet. And I know this makes sense. We're still only twenty-nine. We both need to be ready.

In the darkness, I feel for the writer's bump on his middle finger, the soft knot of flesh raised by years of pens pressed too hard. 'You're going to live a long and happy life, Josh. I promise. I'll keep telling you that until you believe it.'

His grip tightens around my palm, pulse gently pumping. *I know*, his hand says silently.

But he doesn't, not really. And I cannot deny that there is a seed of doubt inside me too. Hard and dark, a tiny stone stuck fast that I can't quite seem to dislodge.

3.

Josh

January 2000

My particular fear of dying has always felt like something and nothing.

Something: not a single male relative in my paternal bloodline has lived past the age of thirty.

Nothing: I've heard the usual arguments a million times. Just a sad coincidence. Doesn't mean it's going to happen to me. The past doesn't equal the future. Etcetera, etcetera.

Some days I can half-believe this. Logic hasn't entirely left the building.

And yet . . . I can't prevent the quicksand fear of it closing in, usually in the middle of the night. I'll spring violently awake, convinced I'm having a heart attack, or a stroke.

As far back as the 1800s, possibly further, every male on my father's side of our family has died young. Not from misfortune, but disease. The youngest was just eighteen. My great-great-grandfather. So in my mind it's long been a case of simple arithmetic, to which the answer is always the same: at an unknown point before I reach the age of thirty-one, my body will malfunction in some way, and I will die.

Whenever these night-time panics descend, I do my best not to wake Rachel. I try to remain still as my heart goes berserk, attempting to recall all the evidence I have for this simply being a phobia.

My GP tried to diagnose me officially, once. 'Thanatophobia, Josh,' she said, with a hint of triumph. As though between us we'd just invented an entirely new subsection of lunatic. 'I believe you have an irrational fear of dying.'

I could have reminded her that my fear, in fact, was perfectly rational. That I had rock-solid evidence running ominously down one side of my family tree. But I'd gone to her for help, not an argument. So I accepted her prescription for anti-anxiety medication, took it for two months, then stopped when it made absolutely zero difference to the way I was feeling.

It happened again this morning, at somewhere around four a.m. The pounding heart. The spasming thoughts. So I got up and went downstairs, stood barefoot in front of a grandfather clock in the huge expanse of the mansion's wood-panelled hallway.

It felt extra-ominous, somehow. Standing in the dark, beneath that sinister wagon-wheel chandelier, surrounded by stags' heads and coats of arms, on a rug made of squashed bear.

Shit, it's January.

This means I have – I am convinced of this – no more than seventeen months left to live.

The masochists are back from their walk. Rachel and I attempt to persuade them we'd simply got the wrong lobby and had been downstairs waiting for them in our wellies all along. We are instantly disbelieved, of course, because Rachel and I are not – have never been – outdoorsy, fond of forced exercise, embracers of mud. I occasionally feel for our imaginary future children, who would no doubt grow up to have rickets, unable to name basic vegetables.

To soothe the collective hangover I cook lunch for all fourteen of us, despite some half-hearted meddling from a mid-comedown Ingrid. Afterwards, Giles talks me into playing cards in one of the many sitting rooms.

I will never not be grateful that my three closest friends all still live within a ten-minute drive of my flat. I know how rare that is – making it through your twenties without one of you relocating to Australia, or moving up north for more square footage, or deciding you've got more in common with new colleagues, flatmates, in-laws.

The sitting room we find ourselves in is more like a library. Floor-to-ceiling bookshelves, every one of them crammed full.

'Reckon they've read all these?' I say to Giles, perusing the spines as if I'm ten again and pressing my nose up to a pet-shop aquarium. The house belongs to a friend of Ingrid's mum, who apparently got rich by renting out a vast portfolio of cheap houses she'd snapped up in the eighties.

'Nah. They're just for show, aren't they? There must be hundreds in here.'

More like thousands, I think.

I picture our flat, creaking under the weight of the piles of books I've read and can't bring myself to part with. They take up every available inch of floor space – the hallway and our bedroom, the living room, my study.

For a moment – fancifully – I wonder if they might have any of my novels in here. That's what I do for work, mostly: I'm a novelist. My debut got picked up when I was only eighteen, the ensuing buzz such that it generated enough cash for a down-payment on the flat where Rach and I live now.

My fourth book was published eighteen months ago. But sales have more or less flatlined, forcing me to supplement my dwindling income with a job teaching creative writing at a local college.

Not that this is a bad thing. The opposite, in fact. It's a privilege, getting to coach someone into becoming the writer we both know they can be. Helping them to craft a complex character or even a simple sentence, and feeling the magic of it land in my spine.

No such alchemy with my own work. I'm trying to write a fifth novel right now, but progress has been pretty dismal. I keep half-starting drafts, then ditching them. Rachel reminds me to follow my own advice: rise at dawn, stay rooted at my desk till dark, re-read all the how-to books I've ever bought. She tells me she knows my next book will be the one.

But none of it really helps. My focus constantly feels off.

I know it's partly the fear, clouding my clarity of thought. A squatter in my amygdala, roadblocking my brain.

Carefully, I pull a book from the shelf I'm next to, flip to the title page.

'Jesus. This is a first-edition *Swallows and Amazons*. It's got to be worth thousands.'

Giles shrugs. 'Take it. They'll never know. Bet they don't appreciate it like you would.'

'Um, I know you're the product of two ardent socialists but isn't that stealing?'

'Redistribution of wealth.' He winks, holds up a port bottle. 'Hair of the dog?'

Thieving booze I can get on board with. I'm pretty sure consumables don't count. They go off, after all, and this library looks as though it hasn't been sat in for the best part of a century.

I nod and slide the book back, though it hurts my heart to do so.

We each take a sofa on either side of a walnut coffee table. The room has that distinctive country-house smell: antiques and dust-choked drapery, beeswax and woodsmoke. I can't quite decide if it's pleasant or not.

Giles hands me a glass. By our knees, the fire spits and crackles.

I raise my glass to his, take a swig, then another. The port is velvet-smooth, but it doesn't seem to soften the stiffness in my stomach. Why can't I relax? Another swig. 'What percentage is this?'

Giles picks up the cards, starts to deal. 'You know, Jeanne Calment smoked and drank her whole life, and she lived to be well over a hundred.'

Is this his backhanded way of suggesting we break into the humidor? 'Who's Jeanne Calment?'

'The world's oldest verified human.'

'What's a verified human?'

'My point is, the people you expect to die early are often the ones who live the longest. Death defies logic, mate. It always has.' He looks up, meets my eye. 'You really believe you're not going to make it past thirty, don't you?'

I could ask if it's that obvious. But I already know it is. It has been for years. Almost as long as he's known me.

I've always thought of myself as rational, but this . . . I just can't seem to shake it. The foreboding that lives in the back of my mind. A crouched animal, permanently primed to pounce.

Giles keeps dealing. 'It doesn't sound like Rachel thinks you're on the way out.'

She says not. And, most of the time, I believe her. Because Rachel is a relentless pragmatist. But sometimes, she gets this look in her eye. A fleeting flash of doubt. A crack of lightning so fast, you question if you saw it at all.

But I guess that's fear for you. It tends to be contagious.

I sip my port, trying to hold on to the image of my wife last night. Our champagne kiss in the wine cellar. The way her brown eyes hooked to mine. How she whispered on caught breaths how much she loved me.

'Maybe you need something big to focus on,' Giles continues. 'Like having kids. They're the best thing we ever did, mate. Truly. Your world transforms.'

Giles and his wife Lola have one-year-old twins, to whom Rachel and I are godparents. My favourite thing is to scoop them up, one in each arm, and talk to them very earnestly about Tolstoy, at which they always get the giggles. And it makes Rachel laugh, too.

Inside me, a splinter of envy lodges. A split-second shard of pain.

Sombrely, the grandfather clock in the corner of the room begins to chime.

'Can I beat you at cards now, please?' Giles says.

I pick up my hand and try to smile.

4.

Rachel

November 1988

I probably fell in love with Josh the very first time we met.

It was November, the year I turned eighteen, and I was two months into university, studying for a business degree. I'd dithered for too long over applying to live in halls, not wanting to leave my dad, and home – even though the university campus was only a few minutes from our house. The equilibrium we'd worked so hard for felt like a spirit level bubble that had only just come to rest.

By the time Dad had managed to persuade me that moving out would be a positive step – the start of an adventure, not the end of everything good – all the halls places were taken, so I was added to the waiting list. Not long afterwards, a room became free.

We virtually collided in the corridor as I was moving in and he was moving out. He was hauling a suitcase behind him, two bags strapped across his chest, weighing him down.

He was dark and lean, a little taller than me. I took in the faded jeans and Vans, the hint of muscle beneath his T-shirt. The soft creep of stubble across his jawline.

'How come you're leaving?' I said, to be polite more than anything else, though I was also secretly hoping to confirm his departure wasn't due to black mould, or some kind of beetle infestation.

'I sort of . . . got a book deal.'

I hesitated, not sure if this was student-speak for something worse than the beetle thing.

He cleared his throat. 'Sorry. As in, I wrote a novel, and a publisher bought it.' His tone was bashful, but I could see electricity in his eyes.

'Wow, that's . . . Congratulations.' Oddly, I almost reached out to touch his arm, as if we were old friends.

In the sterile silence of the corridor, I felt his gaze spread through me. Tiny tributaries of heat, reaching into every part of my body.

'Well,' he said eventually. 'It was really nice to meet you . . .?'

'Rachel.'

He nodded politely. 'Josh.'

And then he hobbled away along the corridor, weighed down by his bags, and I felt a pulse of sadness that he was going.

To my left, a door swung open. Someone stuck a hand out, wrist decorated in bangles, chunky rings on all four fingers. A couple were shaped like skulls.

'I'm Ingrid,' said the slight figure at the end of the outstretched arm. Barefoot in leggings and an Umbro T-shirt, she had ice-blonde hair, but a warm smile and dancing eyes. I noticed a nose ring, a neat slash of plum lipstick.

I smiled back and shook her hand, introduced myself.

'Nice, isn't he?' she said, nodding in the direction of the boy who had just made my stomach spill with stars. 'We're having a party later. Don't worry, I'll make sure he's here. Leave it to me.'

My smile widened. I couldn't help it. 'You don't have to do that.'

'Are you joking? My middle name's Cupid.'

★ ★ ★

Later, at the party in the common room, as I was helping myself to more of the bright red cocktail Ingrid had not only made but invented, Josh appeared at my shoulder.

'I should have left you a list of things to be wary of. And top of it would be any kind of cocktail concocted by Ingrid.' He smiled. 'How's the room?'

'Lovely, thanks. Although . . . you left something behind.'

His face fell. 'What was it?'

I laughed, assuming he was fearing he'd forgotten a pair of dirty boxers, or a porn mag. 'Just a notebook with some poems in it.'

Josh looked as if he'd have preferred it to have been the porn.

'I only read half of the first one, I promise. Just because I wasn't sure if it might be important.'

'Thank God. And no, not at all. The whole thing was an insult to poetry, honestly.'

'Remind me to get it for you later.'

He smiled. 'Thanks. There's bound to be a decent bonfire I can chuck it in on my way home.'

He said this, I assumed, because it was Guy Fawkes that night. But anyway. I didn't agree. I could tell how much longing and love had been poured into even just the few lines I had read.

I started to tell him so, but had to almost shout to make myself heard over the music. Acid house, a relentless, galloping beat. Giving up, I mouthed, 'Hey, do you want to . . .?' gesturing to a sofa at the edge of the room, away from the speakers.

We moved over to it and sat, the cushions sagging slightly beneath us. It was a little quieter in that corner, but only just. We shuffled close together, our heads inclined.

Sipping my drink, which was dizzyingly sweet and violently alcoholic, I asked what his novel was about.

'It's crime. A kind of . . . cold-case procedural thing.'

'Is that the official pitch?'

He laughed, looked down at his hands. I noticed a writer's bump on his middle finger, a soft knoll in the flesh of him. His skin was smudged with ink. I pictured him having ideas for novels in the middle of the night, scribbling them down frenziedly with a leaking pen. 'God, I hope not,' he said.

'You must have worked hard.' I privately envied his bravery, quitting uni after just two months to follow his dream.

He nodded, but modestly. 'Swerved a lot of school discos.'

'Lucky you. I always hated the discos.'

'How come?'

'Two left feet.'

He raised a palm. 'High five to that.'

Our eyes met. His were liquid brown, and I wanted to dive into them. The air between us felt charged, suddenly. Molecules realigning, a shift in pressure.

He asked what my ambitions were, a question I always dreaded, given I could never come up with anything more thrilling than wanting a steady job I might stand half a chance of enjoying. I suspected this lack of imagination would disappoint him. But, equally, I didn't quite see the point of lying.

'Nothing wrong with wanting security,' he said, once I'd filled him in, to my relief. 'I don't think you should ever try to be anything other than exactly who you are.'

At that moment, another friend of Ingrid's, who was having tequila funnelled into his mouth nearby, sat abruptly upright and projected a stream of it directly at Josh. Liquor shot through the air, a surprising volume of it spraying all over his grey T-shirt.

I started laughing, reached out to touch his arm. 'Oh, my God. Are you okay?'

'Sorry, mate,' gasped Ingrid's friend, holding up a hand. 'Sorry. Gag reflex. Sorry.'

Josh just looked at me as he wiped second-hand tequila from his face. 'Gag reflex,' he repeated, deadpan.

I laughed harder. I couldn't help it.

'Do you want to get out of here?' Josh said.

And oh, how I did.

In the distance, just visible in the purple sky above Bedford's building tops, gunpowder was exploding, mingling with the music still beating inside my head. The horizon was hypnotic, whirling with colour and dancing light, the ink of the dark made pale.

Josh turned his body to mine. Somehow, I think he knew he didn't need to speak. Taking my face between his palms, he leant forward and kissed me, his mouth warm and sweet from the lager he'd drunk.

I pressed my back against the cold wall. I could feel his pulse firing. Our skin was hot in the wintry air. The spilt tequila had lingered, the spice of alcohol blending with his ocean-scented cologne. He pushed his hands through my hair, kissing me so deeply that all the breath left my body.

Eventually, he pulled away, levelling his dark eyes to mine. 'I'm really glad it was you, Rachel.'

And I was glad, too. Because – even in that moment – I knew, I knew, I knew.

5.

Josh

March 2000

'I've been talking to Giles,' Wilf says, letting me into his flat one Thursday night.

Wilf is a genius. Certifiably so: once named Britain's brainiest kid, he has an IQ of more than 200 and won a place at Cambridge before he'd even turned sixteen. Back then, the local paper was always running articles on him, and he'd get asked to do things like appear on TV shows to solve maths equations against the clock.

These days, he keeps a lower profile, working as some kind of lab chemist for Big Pharma, earning the kind of salary that still makes his father choke on his own-brand muesli.

'Tea?' Wilf offers.

'Go on, then, if you're having one.'

'I'm not,' he says mildly. But he disappears to make one anyway.

Wilf and I met at primary school. Wilf seems to think he's still indebted to me for stepping in one day as he was being repeatedly shoved against a brick wall by a seven-year-old skinhead. But as I always tell him, anyone else would have done the same.

Perhaps we would never have become friends if that tiny bully hadn't seen Wilf's uniqueness as an excuse to pick on him. But from that first encounter in the playground we have somehow felt loyal to each other in the way that animals do, sharing a bond that seems to transcend any of the usual social norms.

Wilf's flat always reminds me of an art gallery: almost empty, save for a few prominent pieces. Big pleather sofa, bulky hi-fi system and a huge Philips TV. He does have all four of my books lined up on a shelf, though, which amuses me – my entry-level crime novels slotted between hefty textbooks on organic chemistry and the Riemann hypothesis.

He's read everything I've ever written, usually adding his feedback to the margins of my drafts. Rachel does the same, albeit slightly more tactfully and not in all-caps and red pen. Still. I don't mind. I'm pretty sure that, between the two of them, they have made me a better writer.

Weirdly, my fear of dying young was one of the first things I ever confided to Wilf. Or maybe it wasn't so weird. Back then, it just felt like a vaguely fascinating fact I could tell people about myself. A kind of ice-breaker for seven-year-olds. A conversational party trick.

My mum and her relatives didn't see it that way, obviously. They discussed it in grave voices, usually bringing each other to tears, whenever they thought I was somewhere else in the house, or watching TV. And it didn't take me long to understand why. It was alarming how quickly novelty turned into trepidation as soon as I'd given it more than a passing thought.

Whenever Wilf and I discuss it now, his brain usually reverts to its factory setting of statistical thinking. He starts talking about probability outcomes, axioms and risk matrices, at which I mostly try to tune him out. Because it's clear – even with my non-understanding of probability calculus – that the chances of me beating a pattern scored into the sands of time are terrifyingly low.

Wilf returns, passes me the tea, takes a seat next to the fireplace. Outside, a biting March wind is charging the walls of the flat in rips and gusts.

'Giles told me about your problem.'

I sip my tea. 'That all sounds a bit STI-clinic.'

He just blinks at me.

'Sorry – what problem?'

'That you think you're going to die some time within the next—' he glances at his Casio '—fourteen months, two weeks and six days.'

I shiver as he says it. My own personal Y2K, still waiting for me on the horizon. 'This shouldn't be news to you.'

'I meant more that it's imminent. Anyway. I think I may have the answer,' Wilf says, then abruptly gets up and leaves the room.

I just stay where I am, drinking my tea. I have long since stopped wondering if I should follow Wilf whenever he walks off midway through a conversation.

Sure enough, he soon returns. He stands in front of me, hands me a small plastic bag, containing two round white pills.

Gingerly, I take it. Turn it over between my fingers.

'The illnesses that killed your relatives are age-related,' he says.

I frown my disagreement. 'None of them made it past thirty.'

He dismisses this with a headshake. Clearly my contribution to the conversation is not required. 'No – as in, they all died from conditions where ageing is the primary risk factor. Cancer, neurodegeneration, cardiovascular disease, one of the hepatitises . . .'

The words boom ominously, reminding me of those old public information films that used to warn kids off attempting to climb pylons, or playing hopscotch on railways.

'Anyway.' Wilf nods at the bag between my fingers. 'Take one of those, and you don't need to worry. You'll be preserved as you are for the rest of your life.'

My heart begins to pound. 'Excuse me?'

'As in, your body will stop ageing. Instantly. Thereby preventing the diseases that have so far killed off sixty-two point three per cent of your family.'

'What the fuck are you talking about?'

'Don't panic.'

'I won't, if you start making sense.'

'In what way am I not making sense?'

'Anti-ageing pills don't exist.'

'They do now. I invented one.'

I scramble to my feet, drop the bag on to the coffee table as though it burns. 'Why are you fucking with me?'

He looks genuinely crushed. 'I'm not.'

And this is how I know he's telling the truth. Because in all honesty? Wilf would not know how.

We talk long into the night. Twice, Wilf's phone rings. I know it will be Rachel. But for the first time in my life I ignore her calls.

'How the hell does it work?' is one of my first questions. But as soon as he starts talking about cellular senescence and mitochondrial loss and keratinocytes and nutrient sensing – then heads off on a tangent into human cell classification – I have to hold up a hand. 'Layman's terms. Please.'

He bristles. 'I really hate that phrase. The science is the science. Anyway, sorry it's taken me so long. But, as I'm sure you can imagine, it's required quite a bit of refinement.'

My mind is swinging wildly between elation and trepidation. It's making me feel queasy. 'Have you got anything I could drink?'

He makes to take my empty cup.

'No, I mean . . . beer. Or whisky. Or anything.'

He thinks for a moment. 'I have toffee-flavoured vodka.'

At this, I have to laugh. 'Fine. Whatever. Bring it on.'

He hesitates, nods down at the pills. 'Are you going to take one of those? Because I really wouldn't recommend mixing them with any form of C_2H_6O.'

'Don't be a prat,' I mutter, the way I do whenever he feels the need to start speaking scientist.

As he heads off to the kitchen, I just sit staring at the pills. My heart rate must be nudging a hundred. Ironic, I think, if the shock of being told I could sidestep an early death might, in fact, be the very thing that ends up bringing it on.

I'm desperate to talk to Rachel. I know she would have something rational to say about all this. But, right now, my brain is still beetling with too many questions.

'How do you know they work?' I say to Wilf when he returns.

'Pre-clinical trials in the lab.' He hands me a glass containing the novelty vodka.

I take a long swig. It tastes sweet and stupid and is exactly what I need.

'You did this for work?'

'Technically, no. They don't know yet. But I'm thinking about pitching it to them. I mean, I kind of have to, given I developed it out-of-hours in their laboratory.'

'But how do you *know*? Like—'

'Computer modelling. Skin cells, grown from human stem cells. The next step would be sending results to the MCA in advance of clinical trials.'

I try to follow what he's saying. But in all honesty you might as well expect a dog to comprehend a lecture in degree-level astrophysics.

My head is swimming. 'Wilf . . . this could be *huge*. Like, ground-breaking. You could make a fortune.'

He sips his insult-to-vodka. 'I'm aware.'

I mean, he does get paid a fair whack already. We worked out once that it equated to roughly ten times my hourly rate. Still, I don't know anyone who would turn down the chance to become a millionaire if it arose.

Outside, the weather is getting wilder. Rain is beginning to hurtle against the windows. A storm the like of which we haven't had for years. If this flat were a boat, I'd be prepping the emergency flares.

'So, listen. I'd be taking this before . . . it's been properly tested?'

'I've taken one.'

I stare at him, shock sinking through me. 'What? When?'

'A few months back.'

'Why the hell—?'

'It'll work, Josh. Trust me.'

And, in a weird way, I do. I trust Wilf more than anyone else I know. Apart from Rachel, of course.

'Just so I'm clear: I take this, then stay twenty-nine and can't die?'

Wilf laughs into his glass, which is the vodka doing its thing, I guess. 'Well, obviously you can die. If you walk out in front of a bus, or jump off a tall building. But stupidity aside, no. To use your phrase *layman's terms* – your body won't develop any new plaque, or blockages. Malignancies, anything like that. You'll be immune to illness. So, say you take it tomorrow, and your body is healthy – that's how it will stay.'

'Bloody hell,' I breathe.

My mind races back to Rachel. To how terrified I've been, for so long – from the first moment we met, really – of leaving her. How exhilarating it would be, how dizzyingly fucking wonderful, to finally know I might not have to. To be able to live our lives entirely free from fear.

Wilf downs the last of his drink, wipes his mouth with the back of his hand. 'So, do you want them, or not?'

'Them?'

'One for you, and one for—'

Rachel.

6.

Rachel

March 2000

On the anniversary of Josh's dad's death – his twenty-fifth year gone – we go to his mum's house for supper.

A quarter of a century. Twenty-five years of missing out on your wife and son, the life you built together.

Josh has cooked roast chicken, his dad's favourite. When he leaves the table to baste it, Debbie picks up the card I gave her and says, 'This is just so beautiful, Rachel. And I know how much Pete would have loved it, too.'

I drew the two of them in pen and ink from a photograph Josh gave me, Debbie's face upturned to Pete's. We had it framed, and Debbie couldn't hold back her tears when she unwrapped it.

I don't know if natural mothers really exist, but, if they do, Debbie must rank among their best. From the moment we met, she loved me honestly and wholeheartedly, no caveats. I love to watch her with Josh – their shared jokes and easy laughter, how frequently they fold into hugs, murmured terms of endearment. The way she lights up when we walk through the door. I watch it all, greedy for detail, hoping to absorb Debbie's blueprint of mothering, so I can do it the way she does, one day.

In the sugar-soft light of her kitchen, across the scuffed pine of the dining table, she takes my hand. Her brown eyes latch to mine, wide and fearful in a way I have never seen them. 'I'm scared, Rachel.'

Unease eddies inside me. Pete's anniversary is always hard. But it doesn't usually feel like this. As if she's begging me for help.

Her grip on me tightens. 'I can't lose him. I wouldn't survive it. He's all I have in the world.'

It takes me a moment to grasp that she is talking about Josh. And, when I do, I realise the words do not exist to reassure her. Because how can I say, *Don't worry, you have me?* As if that would ever come close to compensating for having lost her husband, and then her only child.

'Does he ever talk about it? With you?'

'Sometimes. He tries not to worry me.'

How much detail do I offer up? Do I tell her about the panic attacks, Josh's middle-of-the-night terrors that have now morphed into a fear of falling asleep? Do I admit that, sometimes, I turn to look at him on the sofa and see his jaw muscle flickering, because he's trying not to cry? Do I reveal that he has made a will, paid into life insurance, stopped making any plans at all beyond June next year?

He has been quieter than usual the past couple of days, seeming distracted, permanently deep in thought. But this isn't unusual as his dad's anniversary nears. A combination of grief, and fear that he will succumb to the same fate, one day.

'Is he scared?' Debbie asks, dabbing at her eyes with a paper napkin. Her hand is warm around mine.

I nod, softly.

'Pete was terrified. He tried to hide it, but how could he not be? When you know that to be your destiny . . . your whole life.'

Josh has told me that losing his father felt like an earthquake. The aftershocks never stopped. Debbie took a few weeks' leave from her job as a radiologist, which stretched into an indefinite career hiatus. Josh said she lost all her appetites – for food, fun, the future. Everything that made her who she was, obliterated by a seismic loss.

Tonight is the first time Debbie and I have ever talked like this, just the two of us.

I can relate to her terror. If ever I allow my mind to stray to the prospect of Josh dying . . . But then I'll always force myself to pick up the phone to Ingrid, or my dad, or any of the people who love me. And they will instantly reiterate that Josh's terrible family history is coincidence, nothing more.

When it comes to Josh himself, though, I have found it is a fine line between reassuring him, and invalidating his fear.

'Rachel?' Debbie says.

'Yes.' I pull my cardigan a little closer around me. It's warm in Debbie's kitchen, at her table by the battered old red AGA. But my skin has gone stiff with goosebumps.

'Do you ever think perhaps you should start a family before . . .?'

She trails off, but the missing words are easy to place. *Before it's too late.*

7.

Rachel

December 1988

A few weeks after the common room party, I found myself in A&E. I was sitting in the waiting room with one eye squeezed shut, trying to focus on anything but the sensation of having had iron filings sprinkled liberally across my left cornea.

After I'd been there a good while, a figure appeared in what remained of my peripheral vision. With some effort, I looked up. And even through just one tear-filled eye, I knew it was – impossibly – him.

Josh had said he'd ring me, as the party wrapped up. So I'd spent the following few days thinking he might call, or maybe come to see me at halls. But then the days turned into weeks. I hadn't wanted to ask Ingrid, not keen to appear needy. So I'd resolved to move on.

And yet. The memory of that dynamite kiss kept tugging me back to him. I couldn't stop replaying our colliding smiles, the flame of his gaze. The magnet of his body pressed to mine. Surely I hadn't imagined it, that forcefield between us?

I was immediately conscious of my mismatched tracksuit and unwashed face. In contrast, Josh wore dishevelment perfectly, endearingly scruffy in loose jeans and a soft woollen sweater, his disordered hair framing those dancing eyes.

Given several weeks had elapsed since our kiss, I felt cautious. Then again, he hardly seemed to be trying to escape me.

'What happened?' he asked, his face etched with concern as he sat down next to me.

'I think I've got something in it.'

'Do you want me to look?'

I shook my head. 'Thanks, but I can't even open it.'

'I'll wait with you.'

'It's two a.m.'

'Night owl,' he said. I could sense rather than see his peat-dark eyes fixed on me. His soft, curious smile. 'Hey, how come you're by yourself?'

I smiled back at him. 'It's two a.m.'

'I came to halls a couple of times.' He cleared his throat. 'And I tried calling. I left messages.'

'Oh.' We had a communal phone, in the bathroom of all places, with a whiteboard next to it. But expecting any of us to be reliable message-takers was always going to be a tall order. Besides, there was rarely space, among the myriad scrawled insults and cock-and-balls sketches and coded orders for mushrooms and weed.

'So anyway, the other day, I kind of . . . wrote to you, instead. A soppy little letter.' He shook his head, as if he couldn't quite believe he'd done it. 'You'll probably get it tomorrow.'

I felt my heart open out in my chest, a tiny parachute. 'What does it say?'

'Ah, I couldn't possibly. I think the mortification would genuinely finish me off.'

Something about the way he said this made me nervous. 'So, how come you're here? Are you okay?'

'Um, it's kind of embarrassing.'

I considered for a minute what he might mean. 'Is it appendage-related?'

At this, he laughed. 'What? *No.* What?'

I laughed too. 'Sorry! I assumed when you said *embarrassing*—'

'—it must be to do with my penis?'

At this, a woman two chairs away huffed, loudly. She was bleeding quite heavily from the temple, which I guessed meant she wasn't in the mood for smut.

I put a hand over my face, letting my hair form a curtain around my rapidly heating cheeks. 'Can we pretend I didn't just say that, please?'

He reached out, gently tucked my hair back behind my ear. 'Absolutely not.'

'Why?'

'Because. You look lovely when you blush.'

Eventually, as dawn was beginning to dilute the darkness, I got seen by a doctor. She diagnosed a scratched cornea, then gave me drops, an eye patch, and precisely zero sympathy for having been clumsy with my contact lens.

Josh got us a cab back to campus, then walked me to my block. Without saying anything, we sat down together on the wall outside.

It was getting light, the sky flaring pink. Somewhere nearby, a robin was singing. The morning smelt of pine needles and frost.

'You never did tell me what you were in for,' I said, after a moment.

He laughed softly. 'Ah. Well, that was actually a strategic decision.'

I nudged him with my elbow. 'Hey, I look like an actual pirate. We're all friends here.'

I immediately regretted the clumsy turn of phrase, because – was it my imagination, or did he momentarily look slightly crushed?

He let out a reluctant breath. 'Okay. Well, I should probably start off by saying I'm not one of those people who dials 999 if they get a splinter or stub their toe. But, last night . . . I thought I was having a heart attack. I mean, I really did believe it.' He stared up at the sky, where the candy-floss clouds were fringing gold. 'I have this weird fear that I'm going to die young.'

'Why?' I whispered.

'Because none of the men on my dad's side of my family have made it past the age of thirty.'

I felt a little simmer of shock. I turned to look at him, my mouth opening involuntarily. 'Including your dad?'

He nodded. 'He died when I was four.'

'That's awful. I'm so sorry.'

I'd never had cause to think I was having a heart attack, but I could imagine how real the fear must have felt. A primal kind of panic – like choking, or drowning. The loneliest kind of helplessness.

Instinctively, I reached for his hand. The world was fridge-cold that morning, but his fingers in mine were warm. And it didn't seem weird, or too soon. It felt just right. I leaned forward, put my lips to his. He responded instantly, bringing a palm to my face. My mouth parted, letting him in for a kiss that was startlingly intense for such a tender beginning. His lips were laced with sugar from the vending machine hot chocolate we had earlier pooled our change to share.

'I would ask you in,' I whispered, as we drew apart after a few moments, 'but, you know. The patch.'

'Is it weird to say I like the patch?'

'Yes, that's incredibly weird.' I smiled. 'It'll be off in a couple of days.'

* * *

Three nights later, I called him to confirm the patch was gone and my squint cured. He asked me to dinner, and suggested Sorelli's, a local trattoria where people queued out of the door for the slow-cooked ragù.

After platefuls of candlelit pasta, and laughing so hard, for so long, that I was risking heartburn, we returned to halls, where I invited him up to the room that had once been his. We were standing by my kettle, valiantly pretending to be interested in drinking coffee, when he turned and kissed me again mid-sentence, as if he simply couldn't wait another moment.

I kissed him back. Seconds began to race. He slid his hands beneath my top, my bloodstream liquid vertigo as his fingers hit my goosebumped skin. He moved closer, pressing against me. The friction felt nuclear. Between my legs, a wet, pulsing heat.

We kissed for a while longer, before I pulled him gently on to my single bed, and slowly, slowly, he reached down to where I was aching and arching for him. And, from that moment on, he was the only man in the world, my orbit, the universe.

8.

Josh

March 2000

We are together in the kitchen when I tell her.

Over the years, cooking has become something of a creative outlet for me, I guess. Especially when I have writer's block. A way of tricking my brain into believing I haven't entirely lost the ability to create things. And it helps that Rachel's a foodie. She spent much of her childhood eating things out of cans, because her dad was working all the time, and they kept shifting between houses. So when we moved in together I resolved to make up for that. My mum taught me young, grounding me in the basics like how to make a really good béchamel, a failsafe Victoria sponge, a crisped-to-perfection roast chicken.

I've been working through the recipes from *The Naked Chef*. I'm trimming artichokes for roasting, rubbing them with lemon. We'll eat them with blackened cod and crusty bread, a chopped green salad, cold white wine.

Rachel is at the table, sketching me. This used to make me slightly self-conscious, the first few times she did it. These days, though, I'm so accustomed to it, I barely notice.

In another life, my wife is an artist. She works at a bank right now, but has sketched in her spare time ever since I've known her. I used to nudge her to take it further. But she has always said she wouldn't want to turn her hobby into work.

As I start to oil the artichokes, Rachel sets down her pen and asks after Wilf.

I let out a tangled breath. I know I need to tell her. In fact, I should have filled her in on the pill the moment I returned from Wilf's flat a week ago.

I abandon the food, wipe my hands, then try to figure out how to put into words the thing that could change our lives forever.

'But they can't be real,' Rachel says, for the fourth time. 'Maybe they're a placebo.'

We are sitting opposite each other at the kitchen table, where I have set down the small plastic bag containing the two white pills. We seem unable to stop gazing at it, as if it's an unexploded bomb.

'Wilf wouldn't lie,' I say. 'He wouldn't know how.'

'So, what, he's been mixing them up in his lab after hours like a mad professor?'

'Essentially, yeah.'

'Using human stem cells? I mean, aside from anything else, ethically, that's absolutely—'

'I know. Ethically appalling. Probably illegal. So he hasn't told his work yet. And he might not, either. Which means we have to keep this between us.'

She nods, slowly. 'But if they've not been tested on animals, or humans, they're essentially unsafe.'

I just have to come out with it. 'This could be my one shot, Rach. It's like looking at . . . a winning lottery ticket. Or a reprieve from death row.'

'Maybe. If you needed one.' She speaks softly, then picks up the bag, turns it between her fingers. 'But you can't risk taking an untested pill.'

'A pill that means you never get old is the Holy Grail. It's what every scientist dreams of inventing. If Wilf can somehow get around being sued, or sent to prison, or struck off the chemists' charter or whatever it is they swear allegiance to, these pills could realistically hit the market in five to ten years. Everyone will want to take one.'

She shoots me a faint smile. 'Everyone?'

'Wouldn't they?'

A tiny headshake to confirm – though of course I should have already known – that she wouldn't be among them.

I try again. 'This pill could save my life.'

She swallows, hard. 'But it could also kill you. Medication goes through rounds and rounds of testing for the very reason that one person . . . I mean, yes, Wilf is scarily clever. But he can't know everything.'

'Can we at least talk about what we do next?'

Her face softens, and she reaches out, grips my hand. 'Of course. Of course we can. God, I can't imagine how impossible this decision must seem.'

I feel my shoulders sink in relief.

She looks down at the bag again. 'How many do you have to take?'

'Just one. That's all you need.'

'Then why do you have two?'

I clear my throat. 'Wilf thought it might be best if we both—'

She drops the bag as if it's stung her, eyes abruptly wide. 'I've never done drugs, Josh. I don't even like taking painkillers.'

'I know. But maybe we shouldn't think of them as a drug.'

In the low light, her brown eyes look almost as if they are burning. 'Okay. Then how should we think of them?'

'A chance to save my life.'

9.

Rachel

August 1980

The thing I remember most starkly about my mother was the void of her gaze. How she would look almost through me, more Victorian portrait than person. So different from Dad, to whom emotion was like good music, to be enjoyed and responded to, impossible to switch off.

Back then, Mum was a roving reporter for a local paper, which meant she always had an excuse to escape me and Dad at a moment's notice.

She and I had never bonded in the way society seemed to deem we should. She appeared committed, in fact, to maintaining the distance that had existed between us for as long as I could remember. So when that summer work trip she went on, the year I turned ten, transpired to be our permanent parting, I wasn't surprised, or even particularly upset. It felt less like a loss than a lifestyle change I could fairly easily adapt to.

But it wasn't quite that straightforward, of course. In the wake of Mum leaving, the difficulties came not so much from her absence as from what it implied. I began feeling scrutinised, sensing that people were judging me harder than they were my mother. Perhaps they were even thinking, *How bad must you have been, for your own mother to walk out?*

Sometimes it seemed that, when Mum left, a strange kind of social angst had replaced her. On sports days or parents' evenings, when Dad couldn't make it and instead I was accompanied by Mum's sister, who – much like Mum – always seemed slightly reluctant to touch me. On Mother's Day, when Dad and I failed to escape the greetings cards and bouquets, the saccharine assumption that all mothers were good. I never knew what to say when people asked where she was, partly because I wasn't actually sure.

Though he tried to hide it, I felt the steepness of Dad's struggle to juggle the parenting and housekeeping and working overtime to make the rent. And he couldn't, not always. For a while we sofa-surfed around Bedford, and I can still recall that life-raft sensation of trying to sleep – or even just relax – in houses where we were always the guests.

'This doesn't define you, you know,' Dad said to me once, as he gently brushed my hair in a bedroom that wasn't my own. 'You are more than what she did. Promise me you'll remember that.'

And so I did. In fact, I resolved to take it with me, always: that I would never make myself accountable for another person's choices.

Reluctantly, Mum did try – I suspect at Dad's insistence, or maybe she felt guilty on some level – to stay in touch for a few years, afterwards.

I remember devoid-of-sentiment birthday and Christmas cards. Awkward phone calls, the odd excruciating visit. On one particularly torturous trip to a freezing and deserted café, where she bought me coffee – even though I'd never drunk the stuff in my life – I asked her why she wasn't coming home. Not to guilt-trip her, or elicit pity. I was just curious, mostly.

For the first time in what felt like years, she looked at me. *Really* looked at me. Her eyes were the tired, dull brown of weathered wood. 'I don't think you'd want that.'

And I thought, *Maybe you're right.*

So perhaps she knew me better than I'd realised.

Once I hit my mid-teens she appeared to lose interest entirely, and essentially vanished for good. And really, I was relieved. Because, to me, forced contact had always felt uncomfortable in a way that no contact at all did not.

As the years passed, Josh and I pondered the possibilities. Depression? An affair? Addictions? Dad denied all these, but perhaps even he didn't know.

Because I just can't believe that feeling nothing for the child you birthed is no more complex than being a bit cold-hearted. I am sure that, even for my mother, it couldn't have been that simple.

10.

Rachel

March 2000

'Well, shit. A pill that keeps you young. Where do I sign?' says Ingrid, setting down three mugs of tea and a plate of buttered crumpets on her coffee table. It is late, and this was unplanned – *Are you free? I need you* – and she is wrapped in a pale pink dressing gown that swamps her slight frame.

'Don't get any ideas,' I mumble.

'You run a wellbeing company,' Polly reminds Ingrid. 'Isn't popping pills against your core values or something?'

Ingrid flicks on a lamp. The room glows gold. 'So's eating buttered crumpets, babe. I won't tell if you won't.'

Polly turns back to me. Her shoulders are damp from the hair wash she rushed to finish when I called, her usually sleek auburn waves now fated to be twice their usual size in the morning. 'And you have no clue where Josh got it?'

'Some kind of doctor.'

It's the first time I've ever lied to my friends, and it doesn't feel good. But Josh asked me to keep to myself – for the time being, at least – that the invention was Wilf's. Not that I would have had the strength of mind to stand between Polly's wrath and Wilf right now anyway.

They exchange a glance. 'Bloody hell. You should get on to the BMA.'

Still Falling For You

I pick a crumpet from the plate and take a huge bite, wipe butter from my lips. 'Not practising.'

I wish I could tell them the truth, not least to confide my fear that Josh will feel some kind of moral obligation to repay what Wilf has done for him by taking that pill too.

Still. Even half a confession feels good. The storm that's been rumbling in my stomach ever since Josh told me about Wilf's invention is beginning to subside.

'You're not going to take it, right, Rach?' Polly asks, her face crumpled with concern.

'She won't even try my home brew,' Ingrid reminds her, through a mouthful of crumpet.

'I mean, I wouldn't, ordinarily,' I say.

Polly takes my hand and grips it, as if we're at the top of a rollercoaster in the moments before it plummets. 'Well, then, you shouldn't. You don't *need* to take it.'

'Maybe I do. Maybe this is the kind of thing . . . Josh and I should do together.'

'Because you're married?' Ingrid snorts. 'If you need something to obey, make it your own instincts.'

'We left *obey* out of our vows, remember?'

'Exactly.'

Polly fixes me with hazel eyes. 'But once you've taken this pill there's no going back, right? The effects would be permanent.'

'Well, yes,' I say, my voice small. 'But so is death.'

Ingrid tuts. 'If Josh really believes he's doomed to an early death, *that's* what you need to address. There's no pill that can fix that.'

I play devil's advocate. 'Look at all his relatives. He can't rewrite history.'

'Okay,' says Polly. 'Maybe we need to be practical about this. Say he does take the pill. If you have kids, when they turn twenty, Josh will be in his fifties. But he'll look like—'

'—he's twenty-something,' Ingrid muses, then nods at me. 'Steady, cougar.'

'This isn't funny. What about when I'm sixty? Josh will look – or be – half my age.'

'Hmm. Might be good for his book sales, I suppose.'

'What? How?'

She shrugs. 'Curiosity sells.'

'Ingrid—'

'I jest. Listen, I don't actually think you should worry. If it came down to it, I'd be willing to bet Josh wouldn't take it.'

I consider this. Perhaps she is right, though I can't deny Josh does have an impulsive streak. A part of his personality that leans into risk, if the weather is just right. His enthusiasm for buying the flat which every expert we'd encountered had warned us not to touch. Some worryingly fearless potholing with Darren in Wales that time. Befriending the particularly aggressive border collie that used to live next door to Ingrid. Agreeing to take a ride in a helicopter flown by a guy seemingly keen to impress Josh's mum, who might or might not have actually been qualified to pilot the thing.

I frown. 'I'm not sure Josh thinks it's that much of a risk, though. Or maybe that's what he's telling himself, anyway. He reckons everyone's going to be taking them soon.'

Polly looks alarmed. In the lamplight, her high cheekbones are gilded gold. 'But who knows what could be in them?'

I'm so close to saying, *I do trust Wilf, in a way*, and only just stop myself.

'Would either of you take it?' I say instead. 'Joking aside.'

'Nah,' Ingrid says, after less than a moment's consideration. 'I'm quite looking forward to getting old. Can't wait to be able to get away with some of the shit my nan does. The woman is *outrageous*.'

I smile, despite myself. The latest story to come out of the nursing home was that Nana Watson had recently feigned what amounted to a full psychotic break just to liven up an otherwise boring Tuesday.

'Poll?' I say, turning to my oldest friend.

'A tablet to preserve me like this? Christ, no,' she says, almost apologetically. 'Might have when I was eighteen, though.'

Ingrid reaches out and takes my hand, which she doesn't do very often, not being predisposed to tactility. I try not to look at the skull ring on her middle finger, the rubies for eyes seemingly trying to find mine.

'The only thing you both need to do now is hang tight,' she says. 'In a year's time we'll be sitting here saying how relieved we are that all this is behind us. Trust me. It's going to be okay.'

11.

Josh

March 2000

A few nights after I tell Rachel about the pill, she gets home from work to find me and Wilf in the living room.

'I thought it might be useful for us all to sit down and talk,' I say, as she pauses in the doorway.

She looks doubtful about this, probably because Wilf's usually a man of few words. He even declined to be my best man because he didn't think he'd have enough to say in a speech.

The flat smells of toast, and the coffee table is covered with empty mugs and piles of paper printouts, as though we've been chairing a council of war. I mean, the past couple of hours have actually been something of a battle for me, on the brainpower front, as Wilf has been attempting to walk me through a paper he's drafted on the mechanics of the pill.

Objectively speaking, his genius staggers me. The potential of this thing. What if everyone took it at, say, the age of twenty-one? How many illnesses and early deaths could be averted? How many lives transformed?

Rachel takes a seat in the armchair near the fireplace. As she does, I notice her mascara is smudged. Has she been crying?

The bank where she works in HR has recently been taken over by a bigger bank with fewer scruples, which means part of her job is now to fire a load of her colleagues and dress it up as redundancy. This, I know, is the kind of corporate savagery that keeps her awake at night. It's got worse since she became a manager last year, which has meant daily full-body immersion into the choppy waters of office politics.

But my wife is nothing if not determined. I know without having to ask that she's going to stick it out.

I meet her eye and mouth, 'You okay?'

She nods, shoots me a little *talk later* wink.

I offer her tea, but she declines, removing her heels and suit jacket, twisting her loose hair into a topknot.

Wilf picks up the book I've been reading from the arm of the sofa. *Jurassic Park*. He flicks through it. 'Interesting choice.'

He knows me too well. 'Coincidence,' I mumble.

Rachel frowns as if she has no idea what we're talking about, which might feasibly be true, since she turned down my invite to come and watch a film about dinosaurs when it was released, in favour of a night drinking pisco sours with Polly and Ingrid.

Wilf dunks a biscuit into his mug of tea. 'Right. I should say from the outset that what we discuss doesn't leave this room.'

'Fine,' Rachel says. Then, 'So, you really took this pill?'

Wilf shrugs. 'I wouldn't expect Josh to be my guinea pig. I had seizures and clots in mind, things like that. Look, in an ideal world the pill would have gone through more rounds of testing at this point, but time's not on—'

I feel my stomach upturn. 'Hang on. You took that pill for me?'

'Yes?' he says, through a mouthful of custard cream.

'Can its effects be reversed?' Rachel says.

She told me the other night, when we finally sat down to eat our cod and artichokes at getting on for midnight, that as far as she was concerned this was the point upon which there could be zero margin for error.

'No. The pill alters the body on a cellular level. There's no changing your mind.'

'You say that like it's not a big deal.'

She directs this at Wilf, but really I know she is speaking to me. To try to remind me. Because she knows that – in the absence of fear – I would ordinarily never contemplate doing something like this.

I've been known to make the odd questionable decision over the years. Ignoring the warnings about our money-pit flat. Bleaching my hair for a dare that time. Strapping myself into a helicopter with that weirdo who wanted to date my mum.

But this . . . this is different. It's funny, what fear can do – the logic it can assign to insanity. Pulling a trigger. Trying to win your money back from the bookies. Freezing on the spot, when in fact you need to flee.

Wilf appears to concurrently consider and reject Rachel's statement. 'Everyone's scared of things they don't understand.'

At this, I have to step in. 'I don't think this is necessarily a brainpower issue, mate.'

'I agree,' says Wilf, sipping his tea and reaching for another biscuit. 'In fact, I was referring to the kind of knowledge commonly referred to as explicit—'

'Sorry, but isn't this all a bit Dolly-the-sheep?' Rachel blurts.

We both look at her.

'Um, what?' I say gently.

'Well,' she says carefully, clearly mindful that Wilf likely feels towards his invention as most people do their firstborn child, 'you could argue it's no different. From cloning a sheep, I mean. It might be seen as trying to play God, messing with the natural order of things.'

'I don't believe in God,' Wilf says. 'And anyway, the creation of Dolly has transformed the landscape of scientific thinking. Her birth indicates that therapeutic cloning is a genuine possibility. Cloning technology could create healthy tissues which could then be transplanted to heal—'

'Sorry – why are we talking about cloning?' I ask.

'People have said the same about every world-changing invention,' Wilf points out. 'The light bulb. The telephone. Bicycles. Penicillin.'

Rachel and I both know we have about as much chance of winning a scientific debate with Wilf as we do of standing on the podium at the next Olympic Games.

But not everything comes down to how big your brain cells are.

The next morning, I wake feeling brighter. Deep down, I know this is because what Wilf has done has given me hope. He's thrown me a lifeline I never thought could or would exist. Now, I might actually have a way out of the early death I have felt so sure for so long is coming for me.

And Rachel is at least willing to talk about it. She hasn't shut it down. I am optimistic, perhaps for the first time, that we can come to some kind of agreement about what to do next.

I wake her with a kiss. I am already showered and dressed, off to work early to prep for class with a coffee on campus.

'I love you,' I whisper.

'Josh?' Her skin is warm from the bed, her eyes still part-drugged with sleep.

'Yeah.'

'Promise me you won't take it without telling me.'

'What?'

Her pupils chase mine. 'The pill. Just . . . promise me you won't take it. Not without telling me.'

'Of course I won't. I wouldn't. I promise.'

'You don't owe Wilf anything. I know he's done all of this for you . . . but you didn't ask him to.'

'I know.'

'Hey, come here.'

I hesitate, stomach twitching. 'What?'

'You have time,' she whispers, with a smile.

'I really don't.'

But even as I'm saying it I'm kneeling over her on the mattress, pressing my lips to hers. We kiss, softly at first and then more hungrily. I keep insisting I have to go, I really need to prep, I'll be late. But the whole while, I am easing away the satin straps of her top, and she is reaching down to feel me, smilingly unzipping my fly, and I am breathing, 'Fuck,' then, 'Wait, wait, socks, socks,' laughing as I kick them off. She flicks my belt undone and tugs down my jeans, the underwear I put on less than ten minutes ago. She sits up, pushes me gently on to my back. Works her way down my body, then closes her mouth around me. I sling my head back and bite my lip, one hand lost in her hair. I tug the duvet into my other fist, shudders of pleasure passing from me to her as I feel myself depart earth.

12.

Rachel

May 2000

'It's the sort of thing my mother would have done, you know.'

Josh prongs a chip with a wooden fork. 'What is?'

'Taking that pill,' I say, flicking a shard of batter on to the shingle for the gulls.

Dad has told me Mum was always trying to jump-start her feelings, endorphin her ennui away. She liked to drink, and gamble. She once bought a stake in a bar – an inordinate amount of money for two people on average incomes trying to raise a child – without consulting my father. *An investment*, she insisted with a jutting chin, which was when the shouting started. Neither Dad nor I were surprised when the whole venture purportedly got mothballed not long after she left us.

Josh and I have come to the south coast for the early bank holiday, to a cosy little B&B right on the beach. We have spent the past two days meandering through cobbled streets, skimming stones across the gunmetal sea, feeling the sting of salt spray on our faces, tasting it on our tongues. We stopped by the town's only bookshop, a crooked Tudor-beamed haven where I was delighted to discover they had copies of Josh's first three novels. I arranged them facing out in a row, covering up the memoir of a politician we both despised. Josh bought an armful of books before we left, in case they'd been watching us on CCTV.

We are sitting on the beach with trays of fish and chips, watching the sun drop through a tangerine sky.

'I had one of those full-body MOTs,' Josh says.

It comes out of nowhere. For a moment, I think he is talking about our car.

'They check everything. Heart disease risk, kidneys, cholesterol ... everything. Anyway, the results came in the post yesterday.'

'And?'

'I'm in perfect health. Nothing underlying.'

In my heart, a chink of light. Nothing underlying means he's not going to die early. He doesn't need to take that pill. He's in the clear.

Maybe this is why he suggested coming away. For a fresh start, a hopeful new beginning.

But I only need to look at him to realise I have gravely misunderstood. I know every nuance of his body language so intimately. What every grade of smile means, each increment of a frown. All the pauses between his words, filled with meaning to no one but me.

'So, now I know my body's healthy ... it's the optimum time to preserve it.'

I feel a jolt of alarm, like waking up to breaking glass at night. 'Doesn't it prove the opposite? That you don't need to take it? This shows they were panic attacks, Josh. You've survived every one of them. It's fear – not your body failing.'

He turns to face me. His skin is burnished copper by the sunset. 'You still haven't told me how you really feel, you know. About taking the second pill. So we both ... you know.'

Stay the same age forever.

I nudge the chips with my fork, decide maybe I've had enough. 'Do I need to?'

'You won't consider it?'

'No, I would. I mean, I *am* considering it. How could I not, if you're saying this is what you want to do?' I frown. 'But still, I can't quite ... picture how it would look.'

'Never having to worry about getting ill, or dying from disease,' he suggests softly. 'Not leaving the people we love. Always having our health.'

I shut my eyes and try to imagine it: being forever in our twenties. Free from fear. A future of infinite possibilities.

But I can't. The vision just won't come. Because my world as it is feels more than good enough.

And yet. What I keep returning to is this: how it could possibly be right, to ask Josh not to take a pill that could save his life?

Overcome by emotion, I lean over to kiss him. His lips are tangy with vinegar. *If you took it and I didn't,* I want to plead, *when would you think we should stop doing this? When I'm fifty? Sixty? Seventy?*

We move apart and he takes my hand, this man I have never not loved, who I trust so deeply, whose judgement I so rarely question.

'I'm not trying to talk you into it, Rach, I promise. I still don't know what I want to do myself. I just ... think we shouldn't dismiss it yet. I want this to be a decision we make together.'

Later, back at the B&B, Josh is sitting on the window seat, the sash raised. I can see stars shimmering, the bright marble of the moon. Sea is sighing against shingle.

'If we took that pill,' I say, 'it would really complicate everything. Starting a family. We'd have to wait, wouldn't we? Until we knew for sure if it had worked, and hadn't harmed us. I mean, that would be the responsible thing to do, wouldn't it?'

He looks back towards me, over his shoulder, dark and brooding. It reminds me of a million pictures I have taken of him. So photogenic, but eternally camera-shy.

But even as he nods, my subconscious is saying, *No, the risk is too great; how do we know if pregnancy would even be an option? And, if it was, how safe would the baby be?*

I climb off the bed, take a single step over to him. I'm desperate for comfort perhaps; I don't know.

He puts his hands to my hips, then nudges up my T-shirt to expose the flesh of my midriff, dipping to kiss it once, twice. His breath is wet and warm against my skin.

'I'm sorry, Rach. I wish I could just . . . not be afraid. I wish we didn't have to think about any of this stuff.'

I lower my lips to his head, drop a kiss into his dark jumble of hair. 'Then let's not. Let's stop talking, or thinking.'

With a nod, he pushes me silently back on to the bed, the mattress so tiny it can barely hold us both. The room is snug enough that we've been colliding with the furniture, and each other, the whole time we've been here. He eases down my shorts, and then my underwear, then his own. And soon he is inside me on a bed that rocks and creaks comically in a way that would ordinarily make us laugh, and perhaps relocate to the bathroom, or, failing that, the floor. But not tonight. Tonight, we make love as though there is something at stake. Breathless and urgent, as you might if you'd just been told an asteroid was on course to obliterate earth. As if it might be the last time ever.

13.

Josh

February 1989

The first time we ever talked about having kids of our own, we'd only been dating a couple of months. Rachel was staying with me at the house I still shared with Mum, who was away for the weekend with my aunt.

Rachel had risen early, sliding out of bed before I was even awake. She told me once she found it impossible to lie still once the day had begun. It was down to guilt, she thought, because her dad had always had to be up at dawn for work.

I paused in the kitchen doorway, as I always did on the mornings after she'd stayed over, watching her wholly absorbed in sketching, or cooking French toast, or warming milk to add to espresso. And I would imagine we were years in the future, that we were living together. Even that she was my wife.

If ever she looked up, I'd yawn and rub my face, as if I hadn't been gazing at her for a couple of minutes already. I didn't want to scare her. Hell, I was scaring myself. It had only been eight weeks, and already I was fantasising about spending my life with this girl.

That morning, Rachel was sitting at the kitchen table, wrapped up in my dressing gown, blonde hair spilling out over the collar. She'd made coffee, in the stovetop espresso pot my mum had been using since visiting Rome with my dad in the sixties.

It wasn't yet light outside. Through the kitchen window I could still see stars, scattered like spilt diamonds across the vault of darkened sky.

Rachel was reading the latest draft of my novel, holding the printed pages delicately by their edges.

'Why did you want him to be a father?' she asked as I sat down next to her.

I leaned in to kiss her. 'Hello. Who?'

'The lead detective.'

Rachel had a knack for this – asking questions nobody else had thought to, not even Wilf, or my agent. She maintained she didn't have any particular career ambitions, but I sometimes thought she might make a good journalist. She was the most curious person I'd ever met.

'I guess he felt more real to me that way,' I said.

'But you don't have kids.'

'You don't think he feels authentic?'

'No ... the opposite. He feels really convincing. I guess I'm surprised you can write so fluently about having kids without actually having had them.'

I smiled. 'My mum gave me some pointers. And there are a fair few kids in my extended family.'

Several moments passed. Rachel sipped her coffee, and I thought again how beautiful she was. Those searching, doe-brown eyes. Her long hair a honeyed tumble against her freckled face. The soft slope of her bones. Cheeks slightly pink from the coffee, pale hands cradling her mug. I couldn't believe how lucky I'd got, to have crossed paths with her mere moments before I left university for good.

'Do you think you'll want kids, one day?' I asked her, as casually as I could, looking down at the table. But I suspected that, in reality, I was fooling no one.

She paused for a moment, even though I guessed she was unfazed by the direction in which the conversation seemed to be heading. The opposite, really. I'd already noticed that one of her very favourite things was getting to know people, understanding what made them tick. How good she was at listening. The most *interested* person I'd ever met. I loved that about her, and I sometimes wondered if it was because of her childhood. Because she'd spent so long with a mother she never really knew.

'Yeah. I really want all that stuff. That's the one part of my future that's always been clear to me.' She turned to look at me, brow crumpled in earnest, and tucked her hair shyly behind one ear. 'Do you think that's weird? After what my mum did?'

'Not at all,' I said softly. 'Doesn't it actually make perfect sense? That you want all the stuff you missed out on as a kid?'

I was speaking from experience. I knew how it felt to fantasise about the kind of life my peers had appeared to take for granted, growing up. How things that were normal – perhaps even boring – to them felt extraordinary to me. Two parents at school plays, sports days, birthdays. Daydreaming in the back seat of the car on long journeys, rather than sitting up front. A third person at home at night, the hum of conversation disguising the tick of the clock.

But Rachel understood all that. We understood each other.

I reached for her hand, rolled her fingers gently between mine. They felt a little cool, in the wintry chill of my mum's tiled kitchen. 'I want all that stuff too, you know. In the future. Some day, once I . . .' But then I trailed off, not keen to muddy the moment with talk of my fated family tree, or what might happen if I were to have a son.

The sentiment was pure, though: I could see myself doing it all with her. The pull of a future together already felt magnetic to me. As natural as an ocean tide, a planet orbiting stars.

She tilted her head, as if something had just occurred to her. 'I love that it doesn't scare you, talking about this stuff.'

I leaned in to kiss her. 'That's because it's you,' I said.

14.

Josh

May 2000

Seven days after our break at the beach, I wake again in the early hours.

The bed sheets are wet with sweat. My left arm is fizzing with pins and needles. My heart is hammering harder than it ever has before. I can hear my pulse rushing between my ears.

I pull myself into a sitting position. Swing my legs off the mattress, perch on the edge of it. Try to steady my breathing.

It doesn't work. I feel it building inside me, a low, cold whistle of panic.

Fuck. Is this it?

I leave the bedroom, head into the hall. Grip on to the dado rail with my fingertips like an old man in his nineties. Ironically enough.

The flat is silent and warm. Claustrophobically stuffy. It is a cloudy night, no moonlight.

You have nothing to worry about.
You've made it this far.
The deaths are just coincidence.
Every test under the sun shows how healthy you are.

Nothing works. Shockwaves of pain begin to spread through my chest, along with an unbelievable pressure, as though I've woken up beneath the rubble of a twenty-storey building.

I know I should call 999. But my overriding instinct is to speak to Rachel. She's away overnight with work, but I just have to tell her I love her, one last time.

But then my breathing tightens again. I gasp with the pain, and the panic.

I have to do something.

I want to live. I don't want to die alone, here in this flat without Rachel.

I don't want to leave her.

I think of my dad, what he would have said. What my mum would say.

Do what you can, Josh. Whatever it takes.

That's what they'd tell me. I am sure of it.

I can't catch my breath. The air feels too thin to drink, as though the flat has been drained of oxygen.

If I didn't before, I know now that I am dying. I am going the same way as every other man in my paternal bloodline.

I stagger back to the bedroom, tug open the drawer to my nightstand, grab the plastic bag containing the pills. Propelled now only by fear, the primal need to survive, I shake one into the palm of my hand.

For a millisecond I stare at it, stiff and white against my shining, sweat-slick skin.

But then the pain unfolds inside my chest again, so I don't think any more. There's no time.

I tip it into my mouth, tilt my head back and swallow.

I have sometimes thought that if relief had a colour, it would be the lavender of the sky at dawn. When you've made it through the night, and you weren't sure you would, there is a certain aching sweetness to the sight of it.

But this morning I can see only dark, violet thunderclouds of regret.

It took less than ten minutes – after my heart rate had returned to normal – for the shame to descend, the guilt of having done something I promised Rachel I wouldn't. I ran to the toilet and heaved and heaved, shoved my fingers against the back of my throat until I tasted blood, trying to bring the pill back up.

Fuck. Fuck. Come on. Come on.

But I was dehydrated. There was nothing in my stomach, no way to force the thing from my body.

I make a strong coffee now – possibly not the brightest idea, given that my heart rate's been on the ceiling for the best part of the night – then return to the living room. I sit bare-chested in my underwear on the sofa, hands wrapped around the cup, trying to think.

My gaze turns to the only wedding picture Rachel and I have up in the flat. We always sort of disliked our official photographs: formally posed and stiff, gazing, as directed, into each other's eyes. Both trying hard not to laugh. It was also the first and only time I'd ever put gel in my hair, which resulted in me looking as though I'd taken a wrong turn out of military service.

But this picture we liked. The sole natural one, capturing a perfect, private moment. We were both laughing so hard that our cheeks were wet, and we were having to hold each other up.

I wish I could remember what had set us off. Rachel can't, either.

The sight of it is like a trip-switch to my heart.

The worst part is that what I have done was entirely illogical, of course. Dangerous, even. Swallowing a substance that essentially freeze-frames your body, in the midst of a suspected heart attack. But, subconsciously, I guess I'd been starting to see that pill as my lifeline. In the thick smoke of the moment, I just wanted to get to safety.

15.

Rachel

May 2000

I am home from my work trip. Josh has cooked, and we sit at our little kitchen table to eat steaming bowlfuls of linguine and clams. I have changed into joggers and an oversized hoodie – both Josh's – my hair loose around my shoulders. I love the feeling of being intentionally unkempt at home, after all the stiff shirts and high heels and hairspray I am obliged to wear for work.

'Sorelli's has shut down,' Josh says, after a while.

Our beloved first date restaurant. 'I saw. Sad, isn't it?'

He nods. 'Feels weirdly emotional every time I walk past it.'

'Slow-cooked ragù till we die.' I smile at him, twirling pasta on to my fork.

He smiles back, but it feels oddly off-kilter, the atmosphere between us strange. Like snowfall in the middle of summer.

Shadows have begun to wrap the room. The water pipes are winding down for the night, clunking and knocking beneath the floorboards. I scrunch my toes, feeling their warmth through my feet.

I notice his battered copy of *Finnegans Wake* upturned on the countertop. A sure sign that he's been attempting to take his mind off something. He's been trying to get through it for the past two years, his go-to book when he needs to distract his brain, because he says he has to concentrate like fuck just to make a single paragraph of progress. Usually, odd as it sounds, I quite like to see that book lying around. Because it almost always results in some creative brilliance, whether literary or culinary. Often both.

'Is it writer's block?'

'Sorry?'

I nod over at the countertop. 'James Joyce has made a reappearance.' I reach across the table and take his hand. 'Please talk to me.' I sometimes have to remind him to do this, when he gets lost in his own head, the thoughts fast and cold as a hurricane, the kind of mental weather that steals your breath.

'Rach. There's something I haven't told you.'

His voice is so abruptly gruff that I stop eating.

'God, this is hard.'

Between my ears, my pulse begins to roar.

They are surreal, these suspended seconds before he speaks again.

'Just tell me,' I whisper.

He steps off the cliff, and I go with him.

'I took that pill.'

I stare at him, and my mouth opens, but no words come out.

Freefall.

16.

Josh

May 2000

I know I need to explain. But short of teleporting Rachel into my head – into that moment, last night, when I was convinced I was dying – I know any explanations I have to offer will fall short.

'I thought I was having a heart attack. I genuinely thought I was going to die.' I lean forward, my arms heavy on the table, linguine abandoned. 'I mean, now it seems . . . But, last night, it felt real. You have to believe me, Rach.'

She doesn't say anything. She just stares at me, with wide, disbelieving eyes.

'All I could think about was survival. Not leaving you. Wanting to live. I kept thinking about every other bloody man in my family and the way they . . . It seemed inevitable. A given that I was going the same way.'

Eventually, she speaks. Her voice sounds blank and taut, not at all her own. 'But that pill isn't designed to save you in the middle of a heart attack. If it works the way Wilf says it does, wouldn't it do the opposite?'

I swallow. 'I know. It was . . . I wasn't thinking straight.'

'So then . . . it can't have *been* a heart attack.'

I look down at the table. The wood is pockmarked with imperfections, little waymarks of our life together. The dent from a stray hammer, courtesy of some bank holiday DIY two years ago. Red wine rings from last Christmas. A scorch mark left by a hot wok, Valentine's Day 1995.

Maybe I will feel relief, at some point. But right now, in the gentle heat of Rachel's gaze, I feel nothing but shame.

We move to the living room and lie flat on our backs, splayed out together on the rug. From this angle you can see all the cracks in the ceiling, the fraying paint, the brown bloom on the plaster where the upstairs flat leaked a year ago.

But, for some reason, flat on our backs on the floor has always been our go-to place to talk. What is it about gazing skyward? An instinctive need to see the bigger picture perhaps, gain some kind of perspective?

Or maybe it is more primal than that. Maybe, deep down, we are all just animals, using the night sky to guide our way.

'They made us do one of those personality quizzes yesterday, at the away-day,' Rachel says, after we've been lying side by side in silence for a while. 'You know: *Do you like networking with strangers? Do you feel more easily persuaded by emotional arguments, or rational ones?*'

On the rug, I turn to look at her. The air in the flat is cool now, and her skin is sprinkled with goosebumps. She is staring straight up at the ceiling, as if she's stargazing, or waiting for a comet that may or may not come.

'Anyway. It said I'm *extremely prevention-focused.*'

I think for a moment. 'Does that mean pessimistic?'

'It means I'm not a gambler.'

I just wait. But I think I know what she is getting at.

'I'd been starting to think that if you took the pill I would have to take it too, if you and I were going to have any kind of future. But I'm not sure I could ever bring myself to do it. I suppose what I'm trying to say is that I'm just not the sort of person who could swallow it and hope for the best. The idea of it being irreversible scares me. And you can't change who you are, can you?'

'No,' I admit. But the truth is, I wouldn't want to change a single thing about the person Rachel is.

She turns her head to mine. The tenderness in her brown eyes feels strangely sharp. 'I'm *happy*, Josh. I love our life. Or I did. I was so excited for our future.'

I shut my eyes against her use of the past tense. Against everything it might mean. The forks and branches of what I have done are starting to streak through my mind now, like cracks across ice.

'I spent my childhood feeling like the odd one out. Like there was something wrong with me. And I can't inflict that on my own children, if I'm lucky enough to have them. I want to be a completely normal mother. The most *boring* mother that ever was. I don't want to still be twenty-nine when they're ninety. Can you imagine?'

I swallow and say nothing. Because – ridiculous as this may seem, given what I did last night – I can't, actually. Aside from anything else, the thought is oddly creepy, on a similar plane somehow to those old guys in Hollywood with girlfriends young enough to be their granddaughters.

It is not the family picture we'd always imagined. Not by a long shot.

'I want to experience *life*, Josh. I want to grow old with my friends. I want to go through adulthood the way everyone else goes through it. I want to bitch about my stretch marks and worry about my pension contributions and tut when I see kids riding pushbikes on the pavement. I've got zero interest in staying this age forever. Do you know why?'

I just wait, still soundless.

Her eyes are brimming with tears now. 'Because all I've ever wanted is the entirely normal experience of growing old with the man I love.'

And, at this, I know – although I think, if I'm honest, I always knew – that it's not going to be as simple as asking her to take the pill too. I was naïve to believe, even for a moment, that it might be.

'I just know that if I took it . . . I might struggle to ever be happy again.'

Her voice is soft, but her words still sting. Snow falling on skin.

I realise, now, that by taking that pill I have stolen Rachel's peace of mind. The person who deserves it the most out of anyone I've ever met.

'Taking it will never be an option, for me,' she says, but sadly, as though she wishes the opposite were true.

17.

Josh

July 1991

On the night Rachel and I moved into our flat in Bedford, after nearly three years together, we lay down side by side on the living-room floor and stared up at the ceiling.

We were surrounded by piles and piles of my books, our clothes, and not a lot else. Because we didn't have a lot else; we were only twenty-one years old. We didn't even have a sofa.

Our friends had just left. We'd supplied the fish and chips, and corner-shop cava, as a thank-you for helping us save on a removals company.

'Do you think they all hated it?' I said, after we'd lain together in silence for a while, adjusting to the sensation of being somewhere new, the syncopation of an unfamiliar neighbourhood. The tap and creak of the overgrown pear tree next door. The sweep of passing cars on the road. Music thumping faintly from different open windows, a disparate, clashing melody.

Rachel smiled. 'Yep. But they don't see what we see.'

'Are you still thinking about that new build? The two-up, two-down?' During our search, Rachel had gravitated towards the many other, more sensible properties out there.

'Nope,' she said firmly, but I was worried she already felt wistful about those smooth walls and pristine carpets, sparkling bathrooms and double-glazing so new it still had the stickers on it.

But my mum had insisted property should be bought with your heart, not your head. Her first house with Dad had been a wreck, she said, and hadn't that worked out all right in the end? (Of course, she skipped over the bit where the place nearly bankrupted them.)

'This flat has character,' Rachel murmured now. 'That two-up, two-down was a beige little box with no soul.'

I smiled, trying not to focus too hard on the water marks streaking like tear stains down the length of the living-room wall. 'Yeah, you can't put a price on soul.'

'We'll make it beautiful,' Rachel said, though admittedly it was hard to know how, given how recklessly we'd ended up stretching ourselves on the mortgage.

Rachel was working by then too, in human resources for a bank. It was an entry-level position, only marginally better paid than I was, when you worked out the equivalent hourly rate.

We lay in the gloom for a while, hand in hand. Our sellers had made the rather absurd move of taking all the light bulbs with them, and we didn't own a lamp. Soon the darkness would swallow us whole.

'We should go and get bulbs,' Rachel said. 'Before the shops shut.'

'They took the curtains, though, too. It'll be like we're on stage.'

She thought for a moment. 'We can put newspaper on the windows.'

I guess, having lived in eight different houses in as many years, she'd learned all the tricks.

'So, how does it feel?' I asked her. 'Having a home of your own.'

I could just make out the shine of emotion in her eyes. 'Unbelievable,' she said.

Still Falling For You

I rolled over so I was lying above her, propped up on one elbow. 'Hey, I've been thinking. I could get another job. While we're doing this place up.'

Firmly, she shook her head. 'You're going to write a best-seller, remember?'

I smiled softly. 'You always sound so sure.'

She blinked up at me. In the darkness, her eyes were tiny tidepools. 'Some things you just know.'

I dipped my head to kiss her. Because she was definitely right about that.

18.

Rachel

May 2000

'Are you sure you don't want me to call an ambulance? You didn't hit your head?'

My father slowly swivels his neck from left to right. 'Fully intact. I told you, it was just a little stumble.'

He's downplaying it now. But he called me earlier, mortified, to ask if I could pop round and help him up off the floor after he tripped on his way to the bathroom.

I make tea and we sit together by the open fire, because today's been unseasonably chilly. Dad's house is a time-warp mid-terrace, all terracotta carpets and flower-power curtains, wood-panelled walls and rattan lampshades straight out of the seventies. To anyone else, aesthetically I'm sure it's mayhem. To me, it represents my father, comfort, home.

I feel Dad watching me over the rim of his cup. He certainly seems okay, if a little embarrassed by what happened. He's in his mid-seventies now, has the white hair and laughter lines to show for it. But his mind and eyes are still diamond-sharp.

'And how are things with you, my darling?'

He asks me this because he knows. Always does, always has.

It is not easy, of course, explaining the concept of the pill to a man who's lived through two world wars and once extracted three of his own teeth because he was too impatient to wait for a dentist's appointment. But luckily Dad has never not taken me seriously. Growing up, I could always rely on him to enter make-believe worlds with me, indulge my imagination, patiently help me pick through whatever maze of overthinking I'd got lost in that day, however trivial it was in reality.

After I've told him, he stares for a long time into the orange flare of the fire.

'We were going to start trying for a family next year,' I say.

'Stability,' he says slowly, eventually. 'That's what children need.'

He has always felt deeply guilty, I know, that he could not offer me this.

'I think a lot of Josh. You know that, darling. But I'd be doing you a disservice if I didn't advise you to consider the direction your life might take if one day you're ... fifty, and Josh is twenty-nine.'

The first afternoon I ever introduced Dad to Josh, at the Cat and Fiddle, they both somehow seemed to sense they could skip over the small talk, not bother with routine pleasantries. They just wrapped their hands around their pint glasses and got straight into the miners' strikes, and Margaret Thatcher, and why Josh had written his first book, and how he'd felt growing up without a father, and the peculiarities of his family tree, and Dad's own tricky childhood in Lincolnshire. Which was classic Josh, I'd already learned, after just a month together. Heart on his sleeve, no pretensions. Years later, Dad told me that, by the end of that first evening, he felt he'd made a friend.

'You know,' Dad says thoughtfully, 'in the end, I did actually grow to respect your mother for leaving. Once some time had passed, I mean.'

Surprised, I lower my cup. He's never told me that before. But maybe, deep down, I already knew.

'She was braver than me, you see. Sometimes, staying means holding out for changes that will never come.

Accepting something that is irretrievably broken, and losing yourself in the process. Sometimes, the healthier thing is to walk away. Sometimes, you leave with love.'

I stare at him, blinking back a hot rush of tears. 'Dad. You think I should leave?'

He takes a long time to answer me. 'I know how much you want to start a family.'

I've never made a secret of it: that, to me, a future without kids would be like a picture with no pigment. Not wholly incomplete, but a sense of something missing, always.

I stare into the fire, watching the flames lick and leap. 'It feels so complicated now. Having kids would feel . . . like a risk.'

Dad nods, then leans forward to take my hand. He smells of spice and vanilla, the same brand of soap bar he has used his whole life. 'Then the only question you have to answer is: do you want to be a mother more than you want to be with Josh?'

19.

Rachel

March 2001

People have always thought it's strange, that Josh and I share a birthday – as if there is something a tiny bit incestuous about it. But when we met, the coincidence felt fateful.

Ingrid disagreed, of course. 'Two Geminis? That's going to be *way* too much.'

'Too much of what?'

'Each other,' she said.

But it never was.

Three months before the day Josh and I are due to turn thirty-one, we are sitting at the bar in the pub at the end of our road when he turns to me and says, 'Rach, we should talk about what happens. If I . . . don't end up making it.' He pulls a small leather-bound notebook from the inside pocket of his coat, pushing it across the bar towards me. 'All the important information's in here. Life insurance, my pension, the relevant stuff about my books, what I want for my funeral—'

'Josh, *don't*,' I say sharply.

Abruptly, he stops speaking, but I do not move to fill the silence. I just take a long swig from my wine glass, and then another, trying to ignore the way my heart is racing.

Eventually, he says softly, 'I just want to make sure you'll be okay. I want you to be prepared. I wouldn't want it to . . . break you.'

I turn to face him, heat speeding to my eyes. 'What are you talking about? Of course it would fucking break me.'

In the gloom of the pub, his gaze meets mine. For a moment we just stare at each other, the shock of our situation reverberating through us all over again.

'You think if you die,' I say, 'I'm going to be worried about finances and logistics and fucking *paperwork*?'

I notice the barman lingering. He's pretending to dry glasses, but keeps glancing at us, obviously trying to work out who's done what.

Josh shakes his head. 'I only wanted to tell you where all the information is. Just in case.'

I grab his hand and grip it, so he knows there is no chance I'm letting him go anywhere. 'We have to stay positive.'

'I'm trying,' he says.

I feel myself soften. The line between dismissal and reassurance is so thin it is sometimes invisible. 'I know. I'm sorry. I know you are.'

Light glances off the watch on his wrist, my gift to him for his thirtieth last year. A Cartier in steel, the most extravagant present I have ever bought anyone. I saved for months, putting aside as much extra cash as I could from working overtime.

Perhaps, on some level, I was trying to say, *This is how much I believe you're going to make it*.

For months now, I have been trying not to dwell too hard on the conversation I had with Dad in his living room last year. I forced my focus away from it, because I had no choice. The only thing I've been able to think about is seeing Josh through to his birthday, in three months' time.

Because of course we are both aware – though we rarely express it in so many words – that there's a chance the pill might not have worked. That perhaps Wilf got it wrong. That even geniuses have off-days. That in twelve weeks' time – or less – we could be facing the unthinkable.

Josh frowns, staring down at the knot of our hands on the bar. 'When my dad died, nothing was organised, and Mum was left with a ton of shit to sort out.'

I take a breath, then slowly push the notebook back towards him. Because doubt is like a disease: once you allow it to take hold, it only multiplies, spreads, infects. 'I promise you, Josh. You're not going anywhere.'

20.

Josh

June 2001

It is our birthday. The day on which I will either turn thirty-one, or fall at the last. It's like Y2K all over again. Only, this time, we're not all in it together.

Until seven o'clock in the evening – the time I was born – I find myself able to do little more than stare at the clock and the seconds inching by, time unfolding in agonising increments.

Rachel keeps reminding me I've made it this far. But by now I can barely speak, let alone think rationally. Until that clock strikes seven, all I can seem to do is pace, fidget, repeat, knowing every breath I take will turn out to be either a blank, or a bullet.

I've been doing some very messed-up maths in my head for a few weeks now, trying to figure out precisely how many minutes it takes for someone to die from a heart attack, stroke, aneurysm. Attempting to pinpoint the *exact* moment at which I might be home and dry. And until I get there, I cannot relax.

Eventually, finally, in the most serene way imaginable, the clock strikes seven. And then one minute past. And then two.

Inside my head, the blood is roaring like a waterfall.

I've made it.
What the actual fuck?
Did that pill save my life?

* * *

A heady mix of euphoria and adrenaline is pinballing its way around my nervous system, and I'm not quite sure how to contain it. So far, I've called my mother and my friends, and left an overly sentimental message on Wilf's machine which I know he will hate and instantly delete.

I go over to where Rachel is still sitting motionless at the kitchen table. The toast we made an hour or so ago, because neither of us could stomach proper food, is cold and untouched in front of her. Usually, on our birthdays, I cook. I make a big deal of it – planning a meal I think she'll love, making my once-yearly trip to our brusque local butcher, buying scallops in shells from the van at the market. I dabble in lemongrass and samphire, burrata and spiced rice. I craft buttery Béarnaises and pillow-soft dumplings, seduce her with dangerous cocktails.

This year, though, I couldn't face doing any of it.

I sit down. Across the table, Rachel takes my hand. Her eyes are shimmering with tears. 'You made it.'

'I made it,' I echo.

I should add, *It's all going to be okay now*. But that feels so far from the truth.

To get here, tonight, was all I ever wanted. Yet, now, it feels infuriatingly anticlimactic. As though I cheated my way to safety.

Which, of course, I did.

'How do you feel?' she asks.

The adrenaline begins to ebb. I let a long breath go with it. 'Weird,' I confess.

'Me too.' And then, 'Why aren't we celebrating?'

Tears begin to clot my throat. 'Because today wasn't just about today, was it?'

She shakes her head. But the expression on her face is odd, unreadable. It's as though she's looking through me. As if she doesn't feel anything at all.

★ ★ ★

Soon after that, she makes her way to the bathroom. When she doesn't re-emerge after ten minutes or so, I go to find her.

'Rach?' I tap nervously against the door.

No reply.

A hot rush of panic hits me. Surely she's not in there taking the pill? Because I know that is not what she wants.

'Rach?' I knock on the door more urgently.

A couple of moments pass, then the lock twists, and she opens the door.

'You're not . . . Are you okay?'

She shrugs softly, tugs her cardigan a little more closely around her. Then she turns to sit down on the closed seat of the loo, where she has obviously been for the past ten minutes. 'Why am I not more happy, Josh?' She shakes her head, rubs her face. 'You're *alive*. You didn't die. We should be fucking ecstatic, shouldn't we?'

I squat in front of her and take her hands. They are limp and unfeeling, her skin cold in mine. 'This is probably normal. I mean, not normal, but . . . understandable. This has all been . . . well, a fucking nightmare, frankly.'

She scans me for a moment, as if she's looking for something she's lost. 'I'm scared.'

'I know,' I say softly. The guilt of having done this to her is a constant cog in my chest, grinding, grinding.

'No, I mean, I'm scared that I'll never feel happy at big moments again. I feel numb right now. Like, I'm not feeling *anything*.'

Dissociation, maybe? A protection mechanism? Her mind shutting down, a hangover from childhood?

'My main memory of my mum is that she always seemed numb, Josh. Even on big occasions. Birthdays, Christmases. Like she'd checked out of life. And I feel checked out right now.'

'You're not checked out. You're talking to me about it. That's *proof* that you're not.'

'I asked her, once, why she used to throw things and drink and scream at my dad. Do you know what she said?'

I just shake my head, wait for her to tell me.

In the slight light of the bathroom, Rachel's face looks sunken and pale, unsettlingly ghostly. 'She said it was because she wanted to feel something. Anything. *Any fucking feeling at all*, she said.'

'Rach—'

'I couldn't bear it, Josh, if I turned into her. I mean it: I don't think I could stand it. Just going through the motions of life. Not feeling the way I'm meant to, at all the big moments.'

'You won't; this is temporary—'

A small, tight laugh. 'But it's not. How we are now is as permanent as it gets. You're going to be twenty-nine *forever*. Nothing will be the same again. The life we'd planned . . . it's gone for good. And I'm worried that a part of me will always be grieving that.'

And when we grieve, we go numb, I think.

I try one last time to reassure her. 'You will never be your mum, Rach.'

'How can you say that?' She gives me the saddest look imaginable. 'I'm her daughter. I'm already halfway there.'

21.

Rachel

June 2001

'I'm not being funny, but when did we start hanging out in churches?'

It's a humid evening, a couple of nights after our birthday. When I left the office earlier, I saw my two best friends standing at the bottom of the steps outside.

'We're staging an intervention,' Ingrid said.

'Into what?'

She slipped an arm into mine. 'What do you reckon?'

'Polly's idea,' Ingrid says now, tipping her head back against the pew we're sitting in, seemingly to examine the stony skeleton of the ceiling.

'Don't knock it,' Polly says. 'Churches are usually empty, they're always open, and there's rarely a chance of anyone earwigging.'

'Except God, obviously,' says Ingrid, with mock solemnity.

Polly shrugs. 'I come and sit in here sometimes, just to get five minutes to myself.'

'To be fair, if nothing else, it's free air-con.' Ingrid sheds her jacket, lets out a serene breath.

'Well, thanks for your concern, but it hasn't come to this.'

She shoots me a look, slides a quarter-bottle of vodka from her pocket. 'You sure about that?'

I stare at her. 'Isn't it illegal to drink in churches?'

Still Falling For You

'No,' Polly says mildly. 'Just a tiny bit disrespectful.'

'It's been a long day,' Ingrid says. 'Plus, Polly diverted me en route to the pub.'

I hold out my hand. 'Fine. Just say what you've brought me here to say.'

She passes me the bottle. 'Actually, we brought you here so *you* could do the talking.'

By her side, Polly nods in agreement.

I told them straight away that Josh had taken the pill, mere hours after he confessed. I turned up on Ingrid's doorstep and she knew without having to ask what he had done. And we've been muddling through the fallout together ever since.

I take a swig of vodka, enjoy the burn. 'I feel stupid,' I confess, after a moment or two. 'Like, maybe it should have been obvious this whole time that Josh wasn't really going to die, just because all his relatives did.'

'That's hindsight bias talking,' says Ingrid.

'Sorry?'

'As in, you think now that you knew all along. But you'd only considered it. You didn't actually *know*.'

'We were staring at the clock for the whole of your birthday,' Polly says. 'I can't imagine what it must have been like for you.'

Somewhere inside, I feel a tiny clutch of vindication. But with it comes a fierce wash of sadness.

At the end of the nave, evening sunlight is streaming through stained glass, spilling rainbows over the stone.

'I keep thinking. About being an old lady, and Josh still being in his twenties.'

Ingrid smiles faintly. 'At least you'll get kudos in the old people's home.'

'Go me.' A beat. 'Long-term . . . do you think we can really work?'

'Anything *can* work, in theory. Look at Rupert Murdoch.'

'What about him?'

Ingrid shrugs, takes a sip of vodka. 'Doesn't he have nearly forty years on his wife?'

I sling my head back and stare up at the arched ceiling, at the lines of medieval bosses marking the passing centuries. 'Oh, you're right. Well, I'll just model myself on him, then, shall I?'

'I mean, you'll kind of have to,' Polly says tenderly. 'If you want to get past this.'

Later, back at Polly's, I ask if I can go up and see the kids, who are all in bed.

Blake, Polly's youngest, is sprawled across his mattress, limbs everywhere, mouth hanging open. I wonder what he is dreaming about. On the balance of probability I'd guess Manchester United. His nightlit room is a shrine to his favourite team, a scarlet blaze of posters and autographed photos, soft furnishings, scarves, signed shirts.

Blake adores Josh, confides in him about all sorts. They always have their heads together if they're in the same room, and Blake will usually kick off whenever Josh has to leave.

I sit cross-legged on the carpet, draw a breath. My dad told me once that he used to do this, after my mother left – just sit on my bedroom floor and watch me sleeping.

'Why?' I asked.

'Just to check you were still there,' he said.

At my back, the floorboards creak. Polly squats down and envelops me in a hug. Warm and soft, a cloak of Chanel No. 5. Ingrid is right behind her.

'I want all this *so* much,' I whisper.

Polly rests her chin on my shoulder, hugs me harder. 'You can still have it. Please don't give up.'

'But I can't have kids with Josh unless I know the pill was a dud.' And waiting to be certain will mean another whole decade, possibly longer, of living in limbo.

Perhaps, in itself, that isn't insurmountable. But the part of me that's begun to pull away from Josh – instinct, or is it something stronger? – feels as if it's here to stay.

'So you wait – what? – ten years,' Polly suggests gently. 'Plenty of people have kids in their forties.'

'But it's a massive gamble, to put it off that long. By the time we know for sure . . . it might be too late.'

'You could do it alone,' Ingrid says.

Polly and I turn to look at her.

She shrugs. 'You don't need an actual partner to have a baby, do you? I've been wanting to remind you of that for ages, but now I'm wondering if it might not actually have occurred to you.'

And maybe this is the moment when clarity finally blows through me, sharp as a winter wind.

I want more than anything to have a family, however that comes into being. But my vision of parenting with Josh has been irreversibly altered by what he did. Our future feels murky and messed-up, like smears across a still-wet painting, the picture confusing now, all its colours strange and wrong.

And I am starting to realise that the longer I leave it to make this call, the harder it will become.

I look round at my friends, and shake my head, just once.

They do not need to ask.

Polly gasps, covering her mouth with one hand. 'Rach. Really?'

'Shit,' Ingrid breathes.

22.

Josh

June 2001

Rachel has gone to Polly's for the evening, so I call Giles, ask if he fancies a drink. Together, we regress somewhat, ending up in a dingy little club called Blackout, to which we have given far too much time and money over the years. It's the kind of place where they don't care if you behave like an idiot, which is lucky for me, since I've decided to hit the dance floor, a once-in-a-decade event. After I fail miserably to moonwalk, Giles wisely retreats to the sidelines, where he observes me with a sort of appalled admiration, as though he's watching one of those contests where people in gazebos speed-eat fry-ups for money.

I can't stop thinking about Rachel. About everything we've shared over the past twelve years. I think of her dad, and what he'll say when he finds out. I think about how badly I've let both of them down.

The DJ starts playing Moby's 'Why Does My Heart Feel So Bad?'

At the bar, someone shoves against me. I snap, shove him back. He swings for me, and only by way of an ungainly but fortuitously timed duck do I avoid having my face rearranged. Giles has to jump in. The bouncers get involved, and – no doubt to Giles's immense relief – the two of us are turfed out on to the street.

We start to walk along the river in the vague direction of home. The surface of the water is pockmarked with falling rain. Bedford's embankment is deserted, the only sound the downpour, and the occasional swish of car tyres in the wet.

'What the fuck was that? Thought we were past having punch-ups in clubs, mate.'

I think this might be the first time in the history of our friendship that Giles has been genuinely pissed off with me.

'I'm sorry.'

At first, he just nods with a tight jaw, before appearing to relent. 'All right. No worries. I know you've been going through it lately.'

I stop walking. The least he deserves, after risking getting punched on my behalf, is a proper explanation. 'Actually, I have to tell you something.'

He frowns, turns to face me. 'Tell me what?'

He staggers to the nearest bench and virtually collapses on top of it, saying he needs a moment to digest what I've told him.

This is fair. So I just sit down next to him and wait.

Rain is hurtling from the sky now, in great, heaving pellets. The air smells earthy, weighted with water.

'What the hell were you thinking?' Giles says eventually.

'I genuinely thought I was going to die.'

'Where did you get it?'

My skin prickles. I can't betray Wilf. Not after everything he did for me. 'No one you know,' I mumble.

'And what does Rach think?'

I picture Rachel, the detachment evident in her demeanour ever since our birthday. She's drifted through the hours, not saying much, even seeming to walk out of rooms whenever I walk into them. It has begun to feel as though she wants to be wherever I am not.

I rest my forehead on my hands. 'I've fucked everything up, Giles. I think . . . I might have broken it.'

'Jesus,' he murmurs, then we both sit for a few moments in silence, getting hammered by the rain. Giles must really be shocked, because he's usually the first to bleat about needing an umbrella if it even threatens to drizzle.

'Rach probably just needs time,' he says, after a while. 'She's a reasonable person. She'll come round.'

'I don't know. Our future looks so different now. All the plans we made.'

He looks across at me. 'Do you regret it?'

How is it possible not to know the answer to that most basic of questions? And yet, I find myself struggling. 'I'm grateful to be alive . . . But this . . . it's fucking killing me.'

'Ironically enough,' mumbles Giles, at which point his phone begins to buzz. He's a project manager for a construction company, and has started keeping a portable Nokia clipped to his belt at all times, in case people in hard hats need to reach him, or a high-rise development explodes somewhere.

Glancing at the screen, he asks me if Lola knows anything. I'm guessing the message is from her, wondering where the hell he is.

I shake my head. 'Just Poll and Ingrid.'

He returns the phone to his belt. 'And you really reckon it's worked?'

I'm sure the true answer is yes, if you take into account Wilf and his unassailable brain. But I tell him it'll be a while before I'm sure.

'I guess the kids thing's on hold now, then?' He rubs his jaw. 'That'd be kind of weird. Them growing old, and you staying like this.'

I let out a long breath. 'Please just tell me what to do, Giles.'

He doesn't answer straight away. In fact, it is an unnervingly long time before he says, 'The only thing you can. Try your best to make it up to Rach, and all the rest ... will be what it is.'

'That sounds worryingly like code for *you're fucked*.'

He stuffs his hands in his pockets, stares straight ahead like he's trying to think. 'Remember when Lo did that stupid poll, at Christmas that time?'

I nod, because yes, it had been pretty stupid. Lola had decided, while a big group of us was hammered, that we should all rank each other – supposedly anonymously, though these things never are – in order of who we thought would get divorced first. Rachel had refused, sensibly. I'd shrugged and put *Lola and Giles* as number one, because she had proposed the poll, so it seemed only fair. Satisfyingly, once the votes were tallied, they came out top.

'You and Rach were voted last,' Giles says. 'Remember?'

I push away an absurd pulse of nostalgia for Rachel and I having tabled bottom. 'It was just a stupid poll.'

'Yeah. But I guess what I'm getting at is ... everyone's always known that you and Rach ... you're solid. There's no chance you won't come through this.'

I appreciate the sentiment more than he can know. But it also makes everything worse, in a way. That I have screwed up the kind of love other people wish they had.

We reach Giles's house first, then I carry on for home alone. En route, I pass a bus shelter plastered with a Lunn Poly advert – a hundred quid off a beach break. The beach itself looks shit, quite frankly. But the image sparks an idea in my mind.

Rach and I have never really been exotic holiday people. Mostly because we've not ever had anywhere near that sort of money. But maybe, right now, a complete change of scenery is exactly what we need.

I think of what Giles said. *Try your best to make it up to Rach.*

I'm not so naïve as to assume a romantic holiday will even come close to sorting out the mess I've made. But I've got to start somewhere.

23.

Rachel

June 2001

I don't have a chance to talk to Josh until the following evening, when I get home from work.

I find him in the living room. He gets to his feet, his expression open and hopeful. Damp-haired, he's freshly showered, wearing jeans and an old Teenage Fanclub T-shirt.

Usually, he would come straight over to put his arms around me. But there must be something in my face tonight that tells him I do not want to be touched.

'I've been thinking,' he says, before I can speak. 'We should go away. Anywhere you like. My treat. Aruba?'

'Aruba's in the Caribbean,' I say faintly.

'Exactly.' His voice is low and earnest. 'Rach, I know I fucked up, I know—'

I talk over him, because I cannot bear to hear the end of that sentence. 'I'm going to stay with Polly for a bit.'

A beat. I watch a lump jump in his throat. 'How long is *a bit*?'

I know now that our world is moments from cleaving in two. The loveliness of our old life, versus a future I never thought I would have to imagine.

'I think . . . we should separate. For a while at least.'

'You're not serious,' he says, after a couple of whirling moments, his face and body stiffening with shock.

I press my gaze to his, so he can be in no doubt. 'I am.'

A muscle quivers in his jaw, and I look at him as if for the last time, his tumbled hair and autumnal eyes, that expressive brow, the gentle contours of the bones in his face.

'Rach, I know I messed up. I know I betrayed your trust and let you down and risked our future and ... But we can get back on track. I want to have kids with you, I—'

'I don't want to wait decades to see if that pill has worked, Josh. I can't afford to. And not knowing what the future holds, for us ... that isn't who I am. Maybe you can live with uncertainty. An unconventional life. But I've felt completely at sea since you took that pill. And I can't live that way. You know I can't.'

He takes a step closer and grasps my hand, as if we're at the edge of a cliff and he's trying to stop me jumping. Through the propped-open sash window drifts the scent of a barbecue, kids laughing on the street, the thump of a football. The sublime simplicity of everyday life. And it reminds me why I am doing this.

A tear slides down my cheek. 'I want to be a mum, Josh. You know that about me. You always have. And I want to be good at it. It already feels wrong, and I can't risk fucking it up. I *won't* risk it.'

His brown eyes parch mine. 'So, what – you're going to go off and have kids with someone else?'

I think of what my dad said. *Sometimes, the healthier thing is to walk away. Sometimes, you leave with love.*

'I want to be happy ... and I don't think I will be, with you. Not now. Not long-term. Maybe we could be, for a while. I'm sure we could pretend that none of this has happened. But everything has changed. And we're going to have to face up to that, one day. And if there's a hard decision to be made ... it will be so much less painful to make it now. Don't you think?'

'No,' he whispers, his voice and whole face crumpling. 'I will never say I think it's the right thing not to be with you.'

24.

Josh

June 2001

Not long after Rachel tells me she thinks we should separate, Polly arrives in her SUV to pick her up. Thankfully, tactfully, she decides to wait outside in the car.

I think I knew straight away that this wasn't an impromptu thing. Rachel doesn't do knee-jerk. It's not who she is. But Polly's turning up feels less as if life as I know it is about to end, and more as if it already has.

From the very first day Rachel and I met, I was afraid of doing something to hurt her. It's why I agonised for two weeks after that party before calling her, or trying to find her on campus. Why I deliberated for a full week further before finally writing her that note.

I know my actions have led us here. But I can't let her go. I can't let *us* go.

'Please stay,' I say again, from where I'm standing in the doorway to the bedroom.

She opens her side of the wardrobe, pulls out a canvas bag I don't recognise. She must have borrowed it from someone. It's the kind of oversized holdall you'd take if you were planning on spending a few months on the other side of the world. 'I can't. I'm sorry.'

'Don't apologise,' I whisper, burning from the sight of the bag. 'Just stay.'

'I love you so much.' She is talking through her tears, voice hopping, almost gasping for breath. 'Which is why I have to go.'

'That doesn't make sense.' I am grasping now. I'm desperate.

She looks at me for a searing moment, eyes hot and brimming. 'It does to me.'

After she goes, I sit on the edge of the bed and stare for a while at her empty side of the wardrobe, the newly bare shelves, the unfamiliar tessellation of my things without hers. Of the two of us, Rachel always accumulated far fewer belongings than me, an inclination left over from her childhood perhaps. She kept actively on top of her stuff, enjoyed some periodic paring-down. But still, our flat is small enough for the slivers of space she has left to seem more like craters.

Outside, light begins to slide from the sky. The flat gets colder. The silence ticks.

I still can't quite believe I am facing my first night without her. That she's not coming back. That this is what she wants.

I know I should call Giles or Wilf, or go to see my mum. Or do anything, really, except what I end up doing, which is to crack open a bottle of whisky and start desperately swigging from it, the way people do when they need to be numb. Trying and failing to soothe my screaming nerve-endings, quell the question that won't stop hurtling around my head.

Why did I do it? Why? Why? Why?

25.

Rachel

July 2001

One Saturday about a month after I leave, I am in Polly's living room, reading *Just William* to her son, Blake, when I hear a hammering on the front door. The rhythmic, insistent fist-thump of someone who won't be leaving till they're heard.

This continues for thirty seconds or so before the shouting starts.

'Rachel? Rach! *Rachel!*'

Fuck. It's Josh.

'Stay there a moment, sweetheart,' I murmur to Blake, then move swiftly into the hall, tugging the living-room door shut behind me.

The hammering – and shouting – is growing louder.

Darren gets to him first. 'Come on, mate,' I hear him say, from out on the front step. 'You're upsetting the kids.'

I almost want to smile. Blake barely noticed the noise, so absorbed was he in the scrapes and adventures of the eleven-year-old rebel schoolboy we'd been reading about.

'You're all red in the face,' Darren says to Josh. 'You're usually the calm one.'

'I just want to talk to her. It's been a month. Please, I *need* to talk to her.'

'She asked for space,' Darren says, but I can hear the apology in his voice.

Darren is right: I have needed space. And I *still* need it, because I know proximity to Josh would be like tugging on the thread that's holding all my doubts and second-guesses together right now. How easy it would be, to unravel every argument I've made for us to stay apart.

But still. It doesn't feel fair, forcing our friends into mediating.

I take a few steps forward, put a hand on Darren's shoulder. 'It's okay.'

Quietly Darren nods and retreats, and I meet my husband's eye for the first time in weeks.

I am not prepared for what it does to me. How even the pull of a thread can cut like a blade.

'You'd better come in,' is all I say.

Darren takes Blake upstairs, so Josh and I can talk in the living room undisturbed.

It's a hot, breezeless day. Josh is bare-armed in a T-shirt, the face of the watch I gave him sparking in the sunlight. Through the open window, the air smells sweet, perfumed by the roses smothering the back of Polly's house.

'You . . . okay?' he asks me haltingly. 'Do you need anything from the flat?'

I hate this, the awkwardness that exists between us now which we cannot seem to shift. *I have kissed every part of you*, I think. Yet here we are – two strangers sitting stiffly in a room, unsmiling on opposite sofas, maintaining a prudent distance, asking polite, pointless questions. *How the hell did we get here?*

I imagine, just for a moment, changing my mind. Disregarding our failed future, sidestepping our quicksand past. Going in to kiss him again, the easiest, sweetest intimacy. I have missed it so much. Josh pushing his hands through my hair, freeing my face. My blood flaming and stomach somersaulting, our want for each other unstoppable.

Fleetingly his gaze meets mine, and I wonder with a drumming heart if he is thinking the same.

But then he clears his throat and says, 'Sorry about the . . .' He raises a fist, mimes banging on the front door.

I shake my head. For this, at least, he doesn't need to apologise. 'It's all right. I know I kind of . . . vanished, for a while. I just thought it would be best if we had some proper distance. It felt like we both needed the head space.'

He nods. 'I know. It's given me a lot of time to think, and . . . I'm angry, Rach. With myself, I mean. I'm angry – and I'm sorry – that I took that pill without telling you. That I disrespected you like that. I'm sorry for not leaning on you more. Because I know I could have done. You never once made me think I couldn't. The opposite, actually. I wanted to call you, that night, and . . . I honestly still don't know why I didn't.'

I swallow, both grateful and sad that he has addressed – entirely unprompted – what has been bothering me so much, these past few weeks. Could I have done more? Did he take the pill because he felt he couldn't talk to me? Is the culpability just as much mine?

Josh rests his gaze on me, dark eyes swimming with questions. 'Rach,' he says softly. 'This was supposed to be a separation. Wasn't it? But it's starting to feel . . . pretty terminal.'

Perhaps he came here today hoping a month might have been enough. But what I have been beginning to realise is that, for us, time is no longer the tonic it once might have been.

'If I'd known you were going to leave—'

'What – you wouldn't have taken it?'

'Maybe not. I don't know.'

My stomach turns to thistles. 'It wasn't up to me to give you that ultimatum, Josh.'

Briefly, he shuts his eyes. 'I know. I know that. I'm sorry. I didn't mean that. I guess I just wish . . . none of this had to happen.'

I resist saying *it didn't*, and look out of the window, at the swifts swooping through the summer stillness. They nest in the pantiles of Polly's roof every year. I adore their trapeze-artist flight, the twisting whistle of their call. Polly says they will be leaving soon for Africa, and I know how empty the air will feel without them.

'It's been good to get some space,' I say.

I see Josh's expression lighten, just a fraction.

'Being with the kids, and Poll and Darren ... it's made me realise what's important.' I am forcing the words out, putting weight behind them, because they do not come easily. 'You chose self-preservation that day, Josh. And I'm doing the same. I sometimes wonder if I'm being selfish, but ... I have to do what's right for me now. Just as you had to do what was right for you.'

He leans forward, rests his elbows on his thighs, rubs a hand through his hair. 'So this is about getting even?'

I let out a flinching breath. 'I know you don't believe that.'

'No. Sorry,' he says softly, quickly.

A moment passes, during which Josh stares down at his hands, his wedding ring, as if taking in for a final time the proof of my once having loved him.

'I didn't want to see it,' he says eventually.

'You didn't want to see what?'

He lets out a fragmented breath. 'Before I came here, I told myself that if you looked happy today – if it genuinely seemed like you'd made the right call – then I would walk away.'

I turn my gaze to the floor, my toes scrunched into Polly's carpet.

'And much as it kills me to admit it ... you do. You look like your old self again, Rach.' His voice cracks and fissures. 'So maybe time away from me has been a good thing, for you.'

I do not look up, because I cannot bear to watch him absorb the fact of it.

'I should go.' He gets to his feet. 'I'll see myself out.'

SECTION II

26.

Rachel

May 2002

Ingrid has surprised us all by falling in love. His name is Sean, and they met a few months ago, at a networking event for entrepreneurs. He's just sold the company he set up in his teens, which was something to do with the ethical importation of coffee beans. He's pretty great: attentive and fun-loving, unwaveringly kind, and excited by her many ambitions.

Ingrid tells me Sean has a good friend who's interested in meeting me.

'Absolutely not.'

'Come on. Why not? This guy's mint, I promise. He sells diamonds.'

I widen my eyes at Polly, who smiles. 'Oh, great. He doesn't sound dodgy at all.'

Ingrid throws a handful of peanuts into her mouth, seeing off a fly with a flattened palm. It's hot today, and our first beer garden session of the year. 'Not out of a van. He's a proper dealer. His family are jewellers. He has his own shop, in Hatton Garden. Come on. One date. What have you got to lose?'

'I just don't feel ready,' I insist.

'Look, in the nicest possible way,' Ingrid says, as delicately as she knows how, 'I'm sure Josh will have been getting back on the horse.'

'Please, stop with the bloody horse.' Beneath the table I slip off my sandals, press my feet into the warm grass.

'Don't worry,' Polly says sympathetically. 'It's not like it's a competition between you and Josh.'

'Why?' I look at her, then at Ingrid. 'Has Josh met someone?'

Yes, it was my choice to leave. But I still cannot picture a day when it does not burn: the thought of Josh kissing someone else, touching her and turning her on, peeling off her clothes. In the ten months or so since Josh and I broke up, I haven't even considered getting to know anyone else. I've only just got used to seeing my finger without my rings and not scrabbling around to work out where I lost them. It still, on so many levels, seems unbelievable to me. Even though I'm the one who left, dating another man would feel like cheating on my husband.

We have spoken occasionally since the day he came to Polly's house. Just logistics, stuff like council tax and redirecting the post. I moved into Dad's for a few weeks not long after that, then eventually found a flat to rent just around the corner from work. It's pretty soulless, in that it looks like a multi-storey car park, and there are lots of passive-aggressive noticeboards in the communal areas, and nobody is ever prepared to make eye contact in the lift. But for now, it is fine. There are three bedrooms, which means I can have people to stay, and I have even set up a tiny studio of canvases in the box room.

Communication with Josh has been made mildly more torturous, though, by the fact that I now have a mobile phone. The temptation to text him throbs constantly, a second pulse beneath my skin. But I know it wouldn't be fair, just because I occasionally get lonely and miss what we had.

So I have promised myself I will keep my distance from him. Especially after what happened last time.

* * *

I've seen Josh in person on just three occasions since last summer. The first, at a bowling alley in October, for Darren's birthday. That night, Polly, Ingrid and Lo acted like my assigned personal security the entire time, so Josh and I didn't even get to speak.

The second was our annual festive drinks at the pub. Josh sat at one end of the banquette, and I was at the other, and, aside from a wordless held glance when I first saw him at the bar, we barely communicated. After that, he got so drunk that Darren had to take him home in a taxi.

But the third time was different.

An old friend of Giles was throwing a housewarming, a few days before Christmas. Giles had assured me Josh wouldn't be there. But a couple of hours in I was exiting the kitchen with a pint in my hand when I collided, quite literally, with Josh. The drink went everywhere, soaking us both.

I couldn't help thinking back to that first-ever party, Josh getting hosed down by projectile tequila. *Sorry, mate. Gag reflex.*

'Shit,' we said, at exactly the same time. And then, 'Sorry.'

After a long, hypnotic moment, Josh reached out to push the ends of my now-wet hair over my shoulder. His dark eyes roved mine. 'You okay?' he murmured.

Five months had passed since we'd been close enough to touch each other. He looked so fiercely handsome that, out of nowhere, a frustrating little film reel began to spool through my mind. Kissing him in cinemas, the backs of taxis. How it felt to be in bed with him, the lightning-strike of his fingers on my skin. Lazy Saturday-morning fucks that stretched almost into Sunday. The weight and heat of him sinking into me.

He was wearing new trainers, olive-green Vans. It was a weird feeling to realise there were already tiny things I did not recognise about my own husband.

Josh let out a breath, as if he was battling a deep urge of some kind. We were standing close now. I detected the woodsy, warmed-earth scent of unfamiliar cologne.

A thought alarmed me. Was the cologne for someone else? And was she here?

My back was against the wall. The hallway was almost entirely unlit, save for some fairy lights sparkling along the dado rail. The hypnotic pulse of trance music was drifting towards us, as though the house had its own heartbeat.

'How are you?' I managed to ask benignly, though my body felt anything but.

'Finally feeling festive.'

I smiled. 'Only now?'

'Well, I watched *Serendipity* yesterday. That kind of . . . got me in the mood.'

For a couple of seconds the moment held. We were hardly breathing, not blinking. Then Josh took a step forward, put a hand on the wall just above my shoulder.

'I miss you,' he murmured, his body a gentle cage now around mine, the watch I gave him for his thirtieth glinting from his wrist.

My heart began to race. I felt a softening between my legs.

'It drives me crazy. Seeing you. Not being able to touch you.'

You can, my heart whispered. *You can. Touch me, Josh.*

'When I'm by myself . . . I think about you.'

Tears rose to my eyes. Hot, salted frustration. *I think about you, too*.

On the stereo, the CD switched to Joni Mitchell's 'River'.

Our all-time favourite Christmas song.

His gaze melted into mine as my heart writhed. In the dark heat of the hallway I felt myself lean forward, the sweet elastic of muscle memory moving me in. Millimetres from touching, encountering again the drug of him, just one last time.

Still Falling For You

And then. Laughter on the stairs. Two people we didn't know clattering down towards us, talking animatedly about foot-and-mouth.

The spell fell apart. Josh shook his head, seemed to collect himself. He took his hand off the wall and met my eye again, but this time only briefly. 'Sorry, Rach,' he murmured, then turned and walked away.

27.

Josh

July 2002

I told Mum about the pill pretty soon after Rachel left. I'd been debating keeping it to myself, worried she would panic about side effects and suchlike. But, in the end, I didn't want to lie to her about why Rachel and I broke up.

She's been doing her best to be brave, periodically assuring me that Rachel will come around, in time. And I think she probably does believe that. She was happy, obviously, not to have had to attend my funeral – as far as Mum's concerned, her only child is still alive, and her family tree's intact for the first time in well over a century. In most people's eyes this would be classed as a solid win. So it's clear she's conflicted, deep down, and who can blame her?

Unsurprisingly, Darren, Giles and Lola weren't too jazzed to find out about the pill a full year after Polly and Ingrid. But they have just about forgiven me. Looking back, I feel thankful they did witness my fear, from time to time over the years. Because I think it helps them to understand why I did what I did.

The weird thing is, I think Rachel gets it, too. Just as I get why she felt she had to leave. Why staying seemed impossible. None of her reasons was lacking in logic.

But in a way this makes it worse. Because I've long been convinced that resentment is easier to live with than regret.

Even a year on, I can hardly bear to be at the flat we used to share. I've been writing a new book, trying to keep my mind occupied. And it has helped, putting words on the page and not actively hating them for what feels like the first time in a long while. The story grips me, but I can't do it justice at home. So I transplant myself to the library and cafés, take on extra teaching hours at the college, where I write between classes. I even head alone to bars and bistros at night, sit there until closing with my notebook and pen.

Rachel and I have yet to do an official division of our stuff, which means I still encounter her every day, all over the flat. I set them tenderly aside, the recipes she tore from magazines, her stockpile of Tunnock's Teacakes, cartoon sketches on scraps of paper. There are tops mingled with my T-shirts in the wardrobe. A half-used bottle of Herbal Essences shampoo I cannot bring myself to smell. An invitation to a wedding, addressed to us both, that Rachel helped design. Her winter coat, still hanging by the front door.

I often think about bumping into her, at that party last year. The way she moved back against the wall, allowed me to pin her there for a few delicious seconds. Her tawny eyes holding mine as our favourite Christmas song came on to the stereo. Telling her I still thought about her, at home alone. The kick of knowing just from her expression that she did the same. How desperate I was, in that moment, to take her by the hand and find an empty room or a bed or a chair, so I could show her again just how much I still loved her.

28.

Rachel

December 2002

One night close to Christmas, I am with work colleagues in a bar for our company Christmas party.

As I settle in for my second drink, I notice Lawrence Carmichael approaching me. He is wearing a Santa hat, a sprig of mistletoe protruding from his pocket.

I know only two things about Lawrence. First, he is on the bank's executive team, and second, he has a reputation.

I hear his name mentioned a lot in passing, like a rumour. We've been in a couple of meetings together before, and it's true he has a kind of stop-talking charisma, the kind I'd usually associate with famous people, or criminals.

He takes the empty seat next to me and swigs from his cocktail glass, staring straight ahead as if we're strangers on a train platform. He is crisply dressed, and there is a certain sharpness to his profile. He is not dissimilar to Josh in appearance, except he maybe has more of an edge – Santa hat aside, obviously.

'What are you drinking?' he asks eventually.

I raise my glass, though it's obvious and I assume he's just breaking the ice. 'Snowball.'

'Very retro. Feeling festive?'

I raise an eyebrow, nod down at the mistletoe. 'You do know I work in HR?'

He shoots me a smile, and I feel it ripple through me. The dark scent of his cologne bites as he inclines his head. 'Hate to disappoint . . . but the mistletoe isn't actually for you.'

I try to laugh it off. 'Just checking.'

'I mean, don't get me wrong: it absolutely can be.'

Even in the gloom of the room, I can see his eyes are startling, the iridescent green of a deep sea in sunlight. I smile and sip from my glass, decide it's best not to respond to that.

'Didn't think you were a Santa hat kind of guy.'

'Well, that just goes to show how little you know me, Rachel Foster.'

I turn to him, surprised. I didn't think he had a clue who I was.

He reclines a little, stretches out his legs. 'I should imagine Christmas parties are a nightmare for you, with your HR hat on.'

'Only if people misbehave.'

I regret this, of course, as soon as I've said it. Because it's already clear to me that Lawrence is not the kind of guy you want to flirt with unless you're sure.

He lets my words hang for a moment, which immediately makes me wonder if I misread his tone. Then he says, 'Heard you did stellar work on the feedback and engagement project, by the way.'

'Did you? Thanks.'

'Sure. Everyone's singing your praises. Talking about our new rising star. You must only be – what? Mid-twenties?'

What a line. I shake my head. 'Very funny. I'm thirty-two.'

Lawrence's eyes widen.

'Please don't,' I say quickly.

At this, he laughs. I can tell he is the kind of guy for whom misconduct is oxygen. 'What? I was going to be nice.'

'Exactly.'

'Meaning?'

'I don't want to have to report you.'

'Report me . . . to yourself?'

Annoyingly, a laugh slips free. I shake my head again, wondering why I am making time to indulge this very strange back-and-forth.

'Out of interest, what did you think I was about to say?'

'Something like, *You don't look a day over twenty-five*.'

'You're wrong, actually.'

I can hardly hear him now above the booming bassline from the dance floor. But I refuse to lean in any closer. 'Really.'

'Of course. That's the kind of thing I'd say to my mother.'

'Okay, then, what were you going to say?' I am cross with myself for asking. For being willing, apparently, to play his game.

He moves his head towards mine. For a surreal moment I think he is about to kiss me. I swallow, my mouth sticky from the snowball.

But instead, he straightens up and gets to his feet. 'Ah, I think I'll keep that to myself. You being HR, and everything.'

29.

Rachel

January 2003

A few days into the new year, I am walking to my car after work when Lawrence catches up with me. It's already dark, the air weighty with woodsmoke and wet with mist.

'Hello, HR. Good Christmas?'

I nod. 'It was nice. You?'

'Sure. I'm one of those wholesome family guys, so yeah. I had a great time.'

I roll my eyes softly, shake my head.

'Fancy a drink?' he says. 'Drown our sorrows. January blues and all that.'

I shove my hands into my pockets, tighten my body against the cold.

'Come on. Let me tempt you to a glass of single-vineyard shiraz.'

'You say that like you think I might know the first thing about wine.'

'Well,' he says, levelling his eyes to mine, 'I could teach you.'

I resist a smile. 'Thanks, but I'd better get home.'

'You have plans?'

'Sort of.' This is true: I was going to add watercolour tonight to a bunch of line drawings I've been working on for my art class. I signed up to it after leaving Josh. In the wake of walking out, I was craving a way to help occupy my mind.

To channel some of my messier feelings into something at least a little beautiful.

Lawrence keeps a respectable distance, though in the foggy car park lamplight his gaze all but pins me down. 'So, in other words, you have nothing on.'

I decide I should probably spell it out to him. 'I don't think us going for a drink would be appropriate.'

Lawrence salutes me softly. 'Aye-aye, Captain Sensible.'

'I have to be sensible,' I say, my breath turning milky in the mildewed air.

'Nobody *has* to be sensible.'

'We work together.'

Lawrence hesitates, then feigns a sudden pain, clutching his chest. A pantomime gesture so ridiculous, I end up biting back a laugh.

'Come on, HR. I think we've had, what, like two meetings together ever? We work in entirely separate functions. Take it from me, I try to stay out of personnel issues as much as humanly possible. Unless they come to me, of course.' Then he reaches out and, ever-so-gently, tugs on one end of my scarf. It is years old, the colour of cobalt, a gift from my dad on my fourteenth birthday. He murmurs, 'Love this, by the way. It suits you.'

In the end, I decide that perhaps I'm overthinking things. So what if Lawrence and I do end up kissing, or even having a fling? It would only ever be that – a bit of fun. Lawrence is hardly the kind of guy you'd introduce to your dad, or your friends. And maybe that's exactly what I need right now.

So eventually I relent, agree to a drink.

By my side in the bar, he looks – annoyingly – very handsome. Shirt sleeves rolled to his elbows, collar open, dark hair just so. His jawline and profile are cut-yourself sharp, his brogues so shiny they actually glint. He fits in well here, in this moody and classy cavern of dark wood and polished brass, surrounded by near-silent serving staff and the watery tinkle of piano music.

'So, Rachel. The last time we were in the same boardroom, I could have sworn you were wearing a wedding ring.'

'What, in one of those two meetings we've had together?'

'Yeah. One of those,' he says, mouth twitching.

'You notice things like that, do you?'

'Not always,' he says, holding my gaze. His playful expression becomes sincere, his green eyes watchful. The devilish glimmer is gone.

This catches me off-guard. I'd been expecting – no, wanting, actually – to come here and indulge in a bit of surface-level flirting. To have a nice time and perhaps get tipsy and forget everything else. I certainly hadn't planned to discuss Josh, who I definitely don't want to think about right now.

I tilt my head. 'Why do you want to know?'

'You're Captain Sensible. I'm Captain . . . Curious.'

'It's complicated.'

'Relationships usually are,' he says, then waits, as though he's sure it's only a matter of time before I am spilling my heart out to him. 'Rumour has it he's a famous writer.'

'A writer. Not famous,' I mumble.

Just before Christmas, Polly told me Josh had got a publishing deal for the book he'd been working on while we were splitting up. She asked if I wanted to join everyone for a few drinks, to celebrate. But, given Josh hadn't even told me the news himself, I declined, convinced he must not have wanted me there. And who could blame him?

'You don't have kids, right?' Lawrence asks.

'Why do you say that?'

He shrugs. 'You're thirty-two. You were married. You don't have them . . . Is there a reason?'

I sling him a look. 'I don't know if you got the memo back in the eighties, but you're really not supposed to ask people that.'

Lawrence, it has to be said, has a very nice laugh. It comes right from his stomach, and feels oddly gratifying, a tiny dart of dopamine. 'Believe me, I get every bloody memo going. But I only asked because I'm interested.'

Maybe he's more perceptive than I thought. It's possible he's good at reading people, has a depth that's easily missed, because I suspect he does spend quite a bit of time pratting about.

I don't know why I decide to tell him the truth, exactly. A combination of the wine, perhaps, and knowing how unlikely he is to ever cross paths with Josh.

'I did want kids. Do want them. Actually, it's all I've ever wanted.' I take another sip of wine, then another. *Ah, fuck it. I've gone this far.* 'But, last year, Josh took an anti-ageing pill, which has left me . . . in a really shitty position, quite frankly.'

This will go one of two ways: Lawrence will either laugh and change the subject, or he'll lean forward and ask more, because he sees that as his 'in'.

Unsurprisingly, he opts for the latter. 'What the fuck is an anti-ageing pill?' He says this with some urgency, as if he's been on the hunt for something similar for years.

Over the rest of the wine, I tell him as much as I know, although I keep Wilf's name out of it. Occasionally, as I talk, I notice Lawrence smiling, as if he's trying to decide whether or not I'm crazy.

But I suspect he concludes it doesn't particularly matter, because eventually, when I'm done, he just says, 'Well, shit.'

'Shit indeed.'

I was hoping I might feel relieved, after telling him all this. Instead, the guilt and resentment of having disclosed private information about Josh tastes faintly noxious. I attempt to wash it away with more wine, sensing Lawrence watching me closely.

'The thing is,' I say, 'I really do love him. Did. Did love him.'

Lawrence doesn't blanch. 'Sometimes love's not enough, though.'

I slide him a smile. 'All right, Plato.'

'No, I mean, I was in a similar situation with my ex. She didn't want kids, and I *really* do, and ultimately we couldn't make it work.'

I study him for a couple of moments, then laugh lightly. 'I'm not falling for that.'

'I'm absolutely telling the truth. Ask her yourself. I have her number right here.' He holds up his phone.

We both know it is the safest of bluffs. 'Well, obviously I'm not going to call your ex-girlfriend and ask her why the two of you broke up.'

He sets down the phone, then takes my hand, looks right into my eyes. My heart begins to pound. His skin feels smooth and clean, the metal of his watch a cold jolt against my wrist. He is looking at me as if the rest of the world has suddenly turned to motion-blur, leaving only the two of us in dazzling, brilliant focus.

'So, what do you say, Rachel?' he murmurs. 'Fancy getting out of here?'

30.

Rachel

January 2003

Lawrence's place feels more like a penthouse than a flat. He's no older than I am, but he seems to have skipped a few rungs on the housing ladder. Every surface is pale and pristine, the marble floors gleaming, all furnishings flawless and perfectly positioned. The space smells of posh candles, the kind of soap you get in nice hotels.

He throws his keys on to a console table, then leads me through to an open-plan kitchen/living area. 'Make yourself comfortable.'

I glance around. His sofa looks stiff, the cushions on top of it stacked three deep. The chairs appear to be almost ornamental. There is nowhere immediately obvious to sink into and relax. So instead I remain on my feet, wander over to examine a painting on a nearby wall. An impasto oil-on-canvas, the colour palette abstract, of a naked woman reclining, her large breasts the unavoidable centrepiece.

'This is interesting,' I say with a smile.

Lawrence turns around, then faintly rolls his eyes. 'My mother's handiwork. She's an artist.' He says this in the same way as you might say *flat-earther* or *egg thief*. 'She gave me that for my twenty-first, if you can believe it.'

'Wow.'

'Yeah, I'd have preferred a watch,' he says darkly.

'You know, I actually sketch a bit, in my spare—'

'More wine?' he says, not appearing to have heard me, crouching to open a silver fridge with a temperature LED above its glass door.

'Sure, thanks,' I say distractedly, leaning forward to re-examine the painting. I have the very distinct and strange feeling that I would love to get to know the woman who painted it, but that's probably just because I've had a couple of drinks.

The interior of the fridge glows a bright aquarium blue. Lawrence extracts a bottle of red, then straightens up and removes the cork.

'You keep red wine cold?'

He starts to pour. 'Actually, certain grapes drink best after a slight chill. But you can't rely on the bars to do it.' He takes a step towards me, passing me a glass. 'Cheers, HR.'

'You know, you don't have to call me that.'

'Don't you like it?' His eyes are fixed against me, green and depthless. I have the vertiginous feeling of almost falling into them.

I bite my lip. 'I don't know. It makes me sound a bit ... strait-laced.'

'Oh.' He smiles, drops his voice to a murmur. 'And let me guess: you're anything but?'

I smile back at him, say nothing.

A kind of soft incredulity creeps over his face. 'Are you nervous?'

'It's the red wine,' I insist. 'I'm famously clumsy. And your flat looks like it would cost a lot to clean.'

'Well,' he says, 'we'd better not risk that, then.'

He reaches out for my glass before I've taken a single sip, setting it down with his, then closes the gap between us, so we are almost touching. His eyes work back and forth across my face, the heat of his gaze turning to helium inside me. 'You have no idea how long I've been thinking about you, Rachel.'

It cannot be more than a couple of weeks, unless he means since well before that Christmas party. But right now I couldn't care less about semantics, because he is taking my face between his hands and kissing me, so intensely it sends little shockwaves through me. Lust rushes my stomach as I respond, running my fingers through his stiff dark hair, marvelling at the foreign feeling of this unfamiliar kiss, the press of this brand-new body against mine.

The kiss deepens, becoming fierce and insatiable, his tongue in my mouth now. The alcohol has turned to voltage in my blood. We move on to the sofa, falling a little awkwardly among the cushions, but our lack of elegance barely registers.

It's not long before he's tugging my top over my head, his full weight pressed against me. My hair has tumbled loose now. He skims my nipples with his thumbs, rumpling the silk of my bra, eyes fixed on my face. I unbutton his shirt, skate my hands across his chest. It is rigidly muscular, mannequin-smooth. He hooks his fingers beneath the straps of my bra, pulls it down, then flicks it off. I unzip his flies, unlock his belt, kissing him harder. I feel a groan pass from his mouth to mine.

So I am about to have sex on a sofa with a colleague, after quite a bit of wine. But it's too late for doubt: my body, with its warp-speed heartbeat, has already decided. Rash and rushed may be the opposite of who I usually am, but this is exactly what I want right now. No, in fact: it is what I *need*. To have sex without feeling sad. A no-strings fuck; pure, undiluted wanting.

31.

Josh

February 2003

The first and only time I've hooked up with a girl since Rachel was last summer.

It wasn't my finest hour.

You'd need a psychologist to unpick what made me do it – because I've not yet been able to, and I was the one making all the poor choices that night – but she was married, I knew it, and I decided not to care.

We met in a bar. She had a jet-black bob and luminous eyes, and a crowd of so many friends around her that they looked like her entourage. I clocked her wedding ring from the off, as well as the fact she was way out of my league. As Darren's twelve-year-old would have said, I was definitely punching. But for some reason she made a beeline for me, then remained at my side all night.

We went back to my flat, where I mixed up a couple of the world's worst cocktails, because she said she didn't like wine.

'Do you do this often?' she asked, once I'd handed over her drink.

I reassessed the cloudy, off-colour concoction in our glasses and shook my head. 'Sorry. Can you tell?'

She laughed softly. 'No, idiot. I meant, cheating on your wife.'

'Oh.' I swallowed, glanced down at the ring still on my finger. 'Not exactly. You?'

'Only when it's worth it,' she said with a glinting smile, then stepped forward and kissed me.

When I think back to that night, I firstly remember the relief. I tried so hard to stay in the moment, to not compare what we were doing with what Rachel and I would have done, as we kissed and touched and eventually fucked. And that was when the realisation finally hit: I could get turned on by someone other than my ex, which I'd been starting to worry might never be possible.

But I also remember the guilt, the next morning. Of knowing I'd had sex with someone else's wife. I wasn't that guy. Or was I so bitter now that I was determined to take a sledgehammer to the happiness of everyone around me?

Seven months on from the world's most unromantic encounter, Valentine's Day rolls around, and as usual the world is shitting hearts. Every shop I venture into seems to be propagating teddy bears and rose petals and love-themed foodstuffs, offering Valentine's-whatever at five times the usual price.

I'm not usually this grumpy about sentimentality. Rachel and I would always enjoy the occasion of Valentine's, in that we appreciated an excuse to cook nice food and drink cava, and have some particularly spicy sex. We'd exchange cards, writing each other sweet messages inside. Rachel always drew hers for me. Sometimes they were hilariously graphic, as if they'd been ripped straight out of the *Kama Sutra*.

When she left, Rachel took all the cards I'd ever given her, over the years. I still have each one she wrote to me too, in a shoebox beneath my bed.

As the day has drawn closer, I have permitted myself to picture what she might be doing to mark the occasion.

Candlelit dinner, new lingerie, new man? None of our friends has mentioned she's seeing anyone. But it's bound to happen, sooner or later.

I last saw her at Darren's New Year's Eve party, a couple of months ago. We bumped into each other at the drinks table. She was glowing that night, gold hair tumbling against her face, brushing the frilled sleeves of her glittered dress. It physically ached, how much I still wanted her.

For some reason, in that moment, I felt an inconvenient need to confess. *I slept with someone else. I'm sorry. It was crap. It meant nothing.*

But instead, I said, 'Rach. I still have the second pill.'

She blinked at me, as if she thought she might have misheard.

It was almost reflex, I think. Because I saw her so rarely now, but had continued to rehearse these conversations by myself in bed, in the shower, at college en route to my classes.

'What?' she whispered.

'I'll keep it for you. In case you want to reconsider. I won't do anything with it. Please, Rach. Just think about it. If taking it would mean that there isn't this chasm between us, if it would change anything for you—'

'Josh,' she breathed, her brown eyes glimmering bronze with reflected party lights. 'What are you talking about?'

There was no stopping me now, apparently. 'I honestly think we've made a mistake. We *belong* together, you know we—'

But at this point Ingrid blustered over to whisk Rachel pointedly away, reducing me to finishing that sentence only to myself, much later that night, once I was home alone.

I couldn't believe I'd said it, actually. I hadn't even been drunk. I already knew she didn't want to take the pill – she'd been clear about that from the start. So why the hell did I think that was the way back to her heart? It made no sense. No sense at all.

Anyway. Most of my friends have plans, this Valentine's. Even Ingrid – who is usually about as sentimental as a surgeon wielding a scalpel – has just moved in with Sean. So I head to Wilf's, because I'm pretty sure he won't feel the need to start talking about Rachel, or ask if I've ever considered speed-dating – the answer to which is no, by the way.

But when he opens his front door he's wearing a Periodic Table apron, looking sweaty and rattled. He's gelled his hair – a lifetime first, as far as I'm aware – then tells me he has a date, and asks if I know how to cook lobster.

Ten minutes later, I find myself in his tiny kitchen, dismembering a crustacean so he can chuck it into linguine. I've only done this once before, with Rachel, and neither of us really liked it, on account of my having clocked the lobster strolling happily around a tank before I paid good money to murder it.

'Tell me about your date,' I say to Wilf, partly to distract my mind from wandering too far down that particular road.

'Actually, I've been meaning to talk to *you* about something.' Wilf leans against his worktop, cheeks rosy from the hob steam. 'Do you fancy investing in the pill?'

I frown, silently apologising to the lobster as I snap off a claw. 'Investing?'

'That's what I said. I've been thinking of pitching the idea to a couple of pharma companies. Maybe including mine. I'm not sure yet. I've registered a business, just in case.'

I know Wilf's had conversations with a lawyer recently. He seems confident he's in the clear as far as intellectual property and ethics and all that other stuff is concerned.

'Thought you might want to put in some of your advance,' he says.

Last November, I got a publishing deal for my fifth novel, a standalone thriller about an amateur detective. It made me feel, in some small way, as if the breakdown of my marriage hadn't completely spelt the end of life as I knew it.

'I didn't get much,' I say, wiping lobster flesh from my fingers.

'Well, don't take too long deciding. You'd need to come on board early doors.' He turns back to the pile of herbs he's massacring with a knife so blunt it's almost bladeless.

'Wilf. Do you . . . still think it was the right thing? Taking the pill.'

He chucks the herbs into a pan simmering with cream, white wine and garlic. 'Why wouldn't I?'

Because, sometimes, I find myself wondering . . . what if I wasn't destined to die young?

The fear of it had subsided in a way I never thought it would, almost as soon as I took that pill. But it was replaced, unexpectedly, by the kind of doubt I hadn't foreseen.

What if all those deaths in my family were purely coincidence?

It's slightly unnerving, stepping back from your problems and watching the light slowly shift. The transformative effects of breathing space.

'Regret is a fallacy,' Wilf states, as though life is simply a series of right or wrong answers, as if we're all just living inside one long, ongoing maths equation. 'You have no way of knowing what would have happened if you *didn't* take that pill. So, actually—'

But then the doorbell sounds its town-hall chime, signalling it's time for me to leave.

'Do you mind going out the back?' Wilf says. 'I don't want her to think . . . you know.'

Deciding not to ask what he means by this, I do as he requests, then stand out on the main road for a long time.

The thought returns to me that nobody has said Rachel is dating at the moment. Maybe I should go round to her place. Ring the bell, just to see if she's there. I could apologise again for having cornered her at Darren's party, for the ill-advised stuff I said. Maybe – who knows? – we would even end up laughing about the fact that it's Valentine's and we're both alone.

I turn in the vague direction of her flat, stick my hand out for a cab.

32.

Rachel

April 2003

I dream that Josh has come to my flat to tell me the pill was just fancy talcum powder, that Wilf butchered the science, that he faked all those Mensa certificates and scammed his way into Cambridge. Lawrence informs him, with a shove to the chest, that it's too late, that we are in love now. He orders Josh to leave.

I wake abruptly, gasping for air as if I've been pushed without warning into a midwinter sea.

It is the third time, now, that I have dreamt this.

I need to call Josh. Just to check it's not real.

But as I sit up, and start to cast around for my mobile phone, I realise Lawrence is also awake. He is perched, fully dressed, on the mattress next to me. This in itself isn't too surprising – Lawrence isn't one for languishing in bed, even at weekends. He doesn't see it as an excuse to talk and touch and kiss, the way Josh and I used to. He's the kind of guy who thinks if you're not up and about by six a.m. you're wasting your life.

He is freshly showered, smothered in his favourite cologne. 'You were dreaming about Josh just now. Saying his name. Over and over.' His dark eyebrows are raised, affecting amusement, though I suspect he's more nettled than he's letting on.

I push the hair from my face, try to work saliva on to my dry tongue. The flat smells pungently of coffee. Lawrence never eats breakfast, just caffeinates until midday.

'Not in that way.'

'Oh,' he says pointedly. 'My bad.'

He has a right to be prickly, I guess. I was on top of him not six hours ago.

I reach out and touch his face – to reassure him or apologise, perhaps both. 'I was dreaming about the pill.'

In the slash of daylight filtering between the curtains, his profile is all clean edges and sharp lines. Sometimes, from a certain angle, I think Lawrence looks almost identical to Josh. But he is much more preened and precisely put-together, even at this hour of the morning.

The sliver of sky I can see is a creamy, wistful blue. It carries the light, dry quality of winter evaporating.

Lawrence sighs. 'Okay, don't freak out when I say this.'

'I'll try.'

He rubs his face. 'Well, I've been thinking. What if that pill doesn't work, and Josh decides he wants you back?'

I feel touched and guilty and caught off-guard, all at once. I shuffle into a sitting position. 'Decides? Like, I wouldn't get a say?'

'Sorry. No, I didn't mean that. It's just . . .' And then he trails off, and looks unsure of himself, which for Lawrence is rare.

'What?' I say gently.

'You're definitely over him?' He reaches out, draws a finger along my bare clavicle. 'Josh, I mean.'

Lawrence is just not the kind of guy who usually needs reassurance on anything. Work, life, sex – you could attack his confidence with a jackhammer on all fronts and fail to produce a single crack.

But then I remember that, in reality, we hardly know each other. So perhaps he's not as infallible as he first appears.

'Do you think I'd be with you if I weren't?' I say softly.

Still Falling For You

'I don't know. We did agree this would be a no-strings kind of deal.'

It's been three months now, but we are still fond of reminding each other that we're just having fun. And it is fun, when we sneak breathily back here to have sex in our lunch hour, or when he sends me deliciously inappropriate emails at work, or when he gives me five minutes' notice for a night out that ends up with us walking home together at dawn, arms wound around each other, pausing to kiss as the streetlights blink off.

I attended a self-improvement seminar at work last week, and it struck me that being with Lawrence does feel a bit like pushing myself out of my comfort zone. Because he is the opposite of me, really – Type A and impulsive and ever so slightly ruthless. He doesn't seem to care too much if people like him or not. Only yesterday I overheard a colleague saying about him, *I refuse to work another day with that absolute weapon.*

So this whole thing does feel slightly audacious on my part. But that is also what makes it – for now – feel right.

I lean forward and kiss him. I am starting to discover, it seems, that Lawrence has layers.

'This neediness is kind of cute, you know.'

He breaks into a smile. 'Fuck off,' he says, laughing, pretending to push me away.

'I'm serious,' I say, going in for another kiss. 'I like this side of you.'

'Yeah?'

'Yeah.'

He fixes his green eyes on mine. 'Well, then, I should probably tell you . . . I think I'm falling for you, Rachel Foster.'

33.

Josh

May 2003

On the early bank holiday, I'm invited to a barbecue at Darren's. It is a perfect spring day, the air clear as water. Acres of blue sky and a still, beating heat.

I try to enjoy the moment, since I've been cooped up indoors for the best part of a couple of months, editing my novel. A self-imposed kind of quarantine, I guess, since every time I go out I seem to feel the urge to deal with my emotions by getting off my face, saying absurd things to Rachel, or doing things like sleeping with other people's wives.

The minute I turned up, before I could even get a drink in my hand, I was roped into playing tag with the kids. But Lo has artfully distracted them now with a paddling pool, freeing me up to take a breather with Darren on a couple of deckchairs.

Which is when Darren tells me – casual as you like – that Rachel has started seeing someone. That she's bringing him here today.

My stomach plunges to a depth I didn't know it had. I glance around the garden, as if the pair of them might already be standing right behind me, feeling each other up next to the rhododendrons.

With perfect timing, a shadow falls over us. I look up, breath catching.

It's only Wilf. But he looks odd. Shaky and pale-faced, as if he's just been first on the scene at a road traffic accident. 'I need to talk to you.'

Frowning, I get up and follow him past Ingrid and Lo, who are dancing to a song by that guy out of *NSYNC, margaritas in hand.

As we come to a pause at the far end of Darren's luridly green lawn, Wilf says, 'I think someone at work knows what I've been doing.'

Momentarily, I'm confused. 'What have you been doing?'

To my surprise, he reaches out with both hands and pushes me in the chest. 'The *pill*, you idiot.'

I stare at him in shock, mind spinning. 'All right. Calm down. What are—'

'Who have you been talking to? I told you to keep my name out of it.'

'No one. *No one*. Only Rachel knows it was you, I swear.'

I did mention Wilf's involvement to my mother, but the odds of her having dobbed him in to his Big Pharma bosses are obviously non-existent. Maybe Rachel's told her dad, because she tells her dad everything. But, even if she has, he is in his seventies and a nice guy, and therefore, I'd guess, an unlikely candidate for shafting his ex-son-in-law's friends.

'Fuck.' Wilf is pacing now. '*Fuck*.'

'What makes you think they know?'

He tells me he's been getting anonymous emails, demanding he share his intellectual property or face legal action. He's been followed while driving home, can hear strange noises outside his flat at night. Has received a few silent phone calls.

'It might be that IP lawyer,' I say. 'How do you know he hasn't—'

'Client confidentiality.' Wilf shakes his head. 'He's way too well thought of to risk that.'

'Okay, okay.' I try to think. 'Well, whoever it is, maybe you should call their bluff. Announce it, officially. Would that be such a terrible thing? I thought you were talking about pitching it, taking it wider?'

He's been quiet on this since Valentine's, other than to say he needs more time to think about it. I'd just assumed until now that he was still feeling sensitive about that night, which he'd ended up spending in A&E because his date turned out to have a previously unidentified crustacean allergy. It's unclear if they've seen each other since.

'I decided against it,' Wilf says. 'I don't want to play God. I'm not comfortable with being responsible for the downfall of humanity.'

At this, I half-laugh.

'Do you think I'm joking?' He glares at me. 'Oh, never mind. I don't have time to explain the socio-economic ramifications of everyone living forever—'

'What are you talking about?' My heart rises to my throat. 'Why the hell did you invent it, then? You told me this pill was a *good thing*.'

Wilf lowers his voice to a hiss, as if he thinks Darren's bird-feeders might be bugged. 'Good for *you* – not for everyone else in the world. I can't have that on my conscience, Josh. I was stupid to even entertain the idea. It was just greed.'

If I were a betting man, I might suspect Wilf has casually floated the idea to his God-fearing parents, of whom he thinks the world.

'Okay, look, let's not panic. I'm sure whoever's doing this is just trying their luck.'

Wilf rejects this notion with his eyes. 'Do you have any idea how much this intellectual property could be worth? They won't just let it drop. I'll lose my job. I could get prosecuted. This is *bigger* than what we did, Josh.'

Still Falling For You

I want to reassure him, because I don't believe anyone could be smart enough to outplay Wilf. We just need to collect our breath, take a little time to think.

But, before I can say any of that, he is gone.

Not long after Wilf leaves, Rachel arrives. She is hand in hand with a tall, dark-haired guy in cargo shorts, polo shirt, Ray-Bans. Darren said before that they work together, and I can see the banker in him a mile off. His feet are hidden by the barbecue, but my money's absolutely on deck shoes.

And, by his side, my wife. In a pale blue dress, blonde hair loose around her shoulders, an early scattering of summer freckles across her skin. She is gripping Lawrence's hand, laughing at something he has said. It must be funny, because her shoulders shake, and she covers her mouth as if he's so bloody hilarious she's about to spit out her lemonade.

I think back to Valentine's night, how close I came to giving the cabbie Rachel's address, after leaving Wilf's flat. But at the last moment I changed my mind. And thank God I did, as I really wouldn't have had the stomach to encounter Lawrence with a rose between his teeth, halfway through doing some kind of creepy naked butler routine.

My heart pounds. *Stay cool, stay cool, stay cool.*

I watch them from behind my shades for a couple of minutes, pretending to be deeply absorbed in what Polly's ten-year-old, Fred, is saying to me about a video game.

I've always loved spending time with my godchildren. But, after it became clear that Rachel and I were no longer going to have kids of our own, the feeling occasionally came closer to bittersweet.

Fred is sketching out what I need to know against a paving slab with his index finger. 'Like, you have a budget, so you have to choose between, like, a police station and a hospital . . .'

Christina Aguilera comes on to the sound system, at which Lawrence extends his hand to Rachel, as though he actually thinks he can pull off grinding to 'Dirrty' right here in the middle of a suburban barbecue.

Aside from anything else, he must not know her very well. Because it's common knowledge among all of us that Rachel would rather die than use someone else's patio as a dance floor.

I realise I can no longer watch. I get to my feet, ruffle Fred's hair. 'Sorry. Got to go, mate. Book me in for SimCity another time, yeah?'

'It's SimCity 4,' he corrects me, with a scowl.

Rachel has moved on, I realise. And, though the thought of it is like a meteor to my chest, I know I need to let her.

34.

Rachel

August 2003

One humid night after work in August, I decide to call Josh.

He left messages for me a few weeks back. But I never returned them, perhaps because I knew he would ask me about Lawrence. And honestly? I had no idea what to say.

It's been over two years now since I left. But my heart is still pre-empting just how hard he will care.

I sit cross-legged on my bed and dial his number. He picks up after only a couple of rings, asks how I am, says it's good to hear from me. I apologise for not getting back to him sooner, and then he just gets right down to it.

'You and Lawrence seemed happy, at Polly's barbecue.'

'You were there?'

'Not for long. I left early.'

I pause. 'Me and Lawrence . . . we're just a casual thing.'

'You don't have to say that for my benefit.'

But the truth is, I am not.

Last week, over dinner, Lawrence handed me a key he'd had cut, for his flat. I must have hesitated when he placed it in my palm, because he shrugged and said, 'No biggie. It's just easier, isn't it, when we're coming and going all the time?'

I knew this was my moment to offer him the same in return. But something held me back. A tiny voice saying, *Tap the brakes, Rachel. Just to check they're still working.* Because, over the past couple of weeks, it's been beginning to feel that this is no longer a fling, or a friends-with-benefits situation – but a relationship.

Commitment doesn't scare me. I want certain things from my future. It's just that I don't feel quite ready to say that Lawrence is the guy I will be doing them with.

But I cannot say he is not, either. It's all very confusing.

After mulling it over for a few days, I had a key cut to my flat too, without telling anyone – not even Ingrid or Polly. I left it in an envelope with a kiss on the front, propped up on Lawrence's desk at the office.

It would hardly be fair to start walking Josh through all these mental gymnastics, though. So instead, I say, 'He's just someone from work. We're having fun. We're not serious, Josh.'

And this – mortifyingly – is the point at which my bedroom door opens.

Lawrence must have let himself in with his key. He's fresh from the office, still in his suit and shoes. But he looks the exact opposite of happy to see me.

'Just someone from work,' he repeats, striding away from me into the living room.

Oh, this is bad. I *know* how bad that sounded. 'Lawrence, I—'

'Well, fuck this.' He grabs his wallet and keys.

I stand and watch him, heart thumping miserably. 'That *is* what we said, though. That we were going to keep it casual. No strings.'

'Yeah, seven months ago, Rachel. And you *know* how I feel about you.' He pauses by my front door, fixing me with simmering eyes. 'It's him, isn't it? That's why you're not divorced yet. You still love him. How many of these cosy little phone calls have you been having?'

'*None.* I swear, you've got it all wrong.'

A slammed-door silence lands between us.

'You know what?' Lawrence says, after a couple of moments. 'You need to decide what you want.'

What I cannot confess, of course, is that, right now, it's hard to know. Because being with Lawrence, I have realised, is a bit like living life on a fulcrum. A feeling of constantly pivoting, non-stop movement in directions I can't always control. The same part of his personality that wakes me with a smile when he's operatic in the shower first thing, and doing six a.m. sit-ups in my living room, is also what has led him to fall out with my neighbours over the pre-dawn motivational music and his insistence on grinding coffee beans before it's even light outside. Compromise doesn't interest him; middle ground may as well be a foreign country.

Mercurial is not usually my thing. And yet. I can't deny being with Lawrence is a low-level thrill. He's never fazed by anything, and can turn me to liquid with just the tug of his smile. He's always trying to make me laugh, even if sometimes the jokes miss their mark. He puts effort into everything, is determined to turn each moment into an experience. And isn't that what life is for?

And the sex is good. Although, is it possible, I recently felt the need to ask my friends, that it's too good?

'What the hell is *too good*?' Ingrid said, bluntly.

It was hard to fully explain. Only that, sometimes, what we do feels a little performative, like something ripped from the pages of a lads' mag. Fucking, not making love. Which is fine, mostly. But occasionally I find myself in seduction mode, flirting a little harder, trying to tease out the foreplay. Weirdly, though, this only ever seems to frustrate him, not turn him on.

It could have gone better, too, when I introduced him to Polly and Ingrid, who are not easily charmed. Lawrence expressed surprise that Polly had had her kids so young, telling me later he'd intended it as a compliment. He then asked Ingrid about her company turnover, responding to her answer by saying, 'Well done you.'

Sometimes, all this stuff feels like tiny red flags fluttering in my gut, ones I know I shouldn't ignore.

'Maybe we should take a step back,' I whisper to him now. 'I'm sorry. I'm just not sure I'm ready for this.'

'Didn't you leave your husband because you wanted kids?'

Perspiration is beading on my skin. The flat is hot, humming with trapped summer heat. 'That isn't—'

'So am I not good enough?' He spreads his arms. 'What is this – some kind of fucking audition process for the father of your child?'

'Lawrence,' I say, surprised. 'We're nowhere near—'

'No. But we could be.' He steps forward, voice trembling. He really is hurting, I realise. 'You and me . . . we could be so good. We want the same things. We could have a great life together. You're holding back over nothing.'

I swallow, feeling sweat sliding down between my shoulder blades.

'I love you,' he says, eyes glassy with emotion.

It is not the first time he has said this to me. But, so far, I have not said it back.

'Right,' he whispers softly, eventually. 'Well, that couldn't be any clearer, could it?'

35.

Rachel

August 2003

Ingrid takes me out for cocktails, demands to know why I've been so morose of late.

After I tell her what happened with Lawrence, she looks me dead in the eye and says, 'I've been wanting to say this to you for a while, babe.'

For maybe the first time in my life, I find I do not want to hear the truth from Ingrid. Already I am flinching from the fear of what she might say.

'Lawrence is a love-bomber.'

'A what?'

'You know: he'll shower you with attention and affection until you let your guard down. And then he'll be off. Nowhere to be seen. Speck of dust on the horizon. Classic.'

'Classic what?' I say doubtfully, thinking unexpectedly of my mother. I wonder if maybe she was a love-bomber, when she first met my dad.

Ingrid eyes me over the top of her negroni. 'Just be careful,' is all she says.

Last night, I went to see my father. He asked after Lawrence, so I ended up telling him, as well, what had happened between us.

I'd expected Dad might express some paternal wariness about Lawrence expecting too much, too soon. But instead, he surprised me by saying, 'You need to move on from Josh, sweetheart. You chose to leave him so you could have a future.'

'Right,' I said uncertainly, even as I was thinking, *But you loved Josh, Dad.*

He spread his hands, wise old Dad, dispensing sage advice in his dressing gown from his fireside armchair. 'So, it would be illogical to let Josh stop that from happening. Wouldn't it?'

Two weeks pass. Lawrence doesn't call, or text. His office is empty whenever I walk past it at work, and he hasn't responded to any of my tentative emails to him either.

One night, though, I am working late when I notice his office light is on. It has been dark and deserted all day, so I guess he's just returned from meetings off-site somewhere.

I take a breath, then leave my cubicle and go to knock on his door.

He looks up. He is sitting behind his desk, tie loose, tapping on the upgraded Nokia work gave him last month.

Through the glass, our eyes meet.

He doesn't smile. But he does beckon me in.

'What's this?' he says with a sigh, when I set a bottle bag on his desk. I've had it with me for a couple of days, waiting for the right moment to give it to him.

'Single-vineyard shiraz. I'm reliably informed it's a good one.'

It cost more than I've spent on a bottle of wine in my entire life. Not that it's about the money. But I do want him to know how sorry I am.

He folds his arms, settles back in his chair, doesn't go near the bag. 'Yeah? What's the occasion?'

'The occasion of me wanting to make it up to you. I am sorry, Lawrence.'

Silence spills through the room. Neither of us moves.

Eventually, he says, 'Do you have your HR hat on right now, HR?'

I smile cautiously. 'Nope.'

He nods down at the bottle. 'Better crack that open, then.'

We drink wine by the light of his desk lamp. The whole building is silent, save for the faint whirr of static from idling photocopiers. Beyond the glass doors of Lawrence's office, the rest of the vast space is an open ocean of black.

Lawrence still has one of those giant leather-edged ink blotters, even though I don't think I've ever seen him write with a fountain pen. Behind his desk, there are lots of framed training certificates for things like capital markets and financial modelling, operational risk.

He follows my eye, smiling faintly. 'I get jealous, sometimes. Of all the guys here with framed photos of their wives and kids on their desks. A solid pass in preventing financial crime isn't quite the same, is it?'

I have really missed you, I think. It surprised me, actually, when we stopped speaking, just how hard his absence hit. Like going cold turkey from a drug you didn't know you were hooked on.

'Lawrence . . .' I say.

He nods once, then waits.

'I obviously don't see you as "just" someone from the office.'

'Is it obvious, though?' His green eyes are a jungle, dark and impenetrable. 'I mean, that is what you said, when you thought I wasn't listening.'

He's not about to make this easy on me, which is fair enough. 'I was protecting Josh's feelings.'

Tilting his glass to the light, he takes a long sip. 'Why?'

I swallow. I promised myself before I came in here that I would be as honest as I could. 'We were married . . . I guess it felt like a sensitive subject. And you and me . . . It's taken me time to adjust, to the idea of being in a serious relationship again. Because we did always say we were just having fun. Not swapping keys, and saying *I love you* and—'

'Rachel, don't get me wrong,' Lawrence says, leaning forward in his swivel chair, fixing me with earnest eyes. 'I was more surprised than anyone when I realised I was having those feelings for you. But don't you think that means it's real? Isn't that the most pure kind of emotion there is? Something that appears out of nowhere? That catches you completely off-guard?'

I wonder if I agree, or if Lawrence is in fact talking about lust. A commotion of chemicals, our body's way of bypassing our brains. Wilf lectured us all about this once over dinner, only piping down when Ingrid snapped a breadstick in half and lobbed both pieces at his head.

'We can *be* something, Rachel,' Lawrence insists. 'I know we can.'

He gets to his feet, comes round to my side of the desk and bends down to kiss me, murmuring, 'God, I've missed you so much.' He tips my face up between his hands. I part my lips, let him in. His mouth is supple and smoky from the wine, the kiss so vigorous it feels almost territorial, and my heart is going berserk now and all the chemicals Wilf was talking about are shooting through my bloodstream, and I think, *Fuck it, and fuck you, Wilf, and your bullshit dopamine cocktail theories. Lawrence is right – this is too good,* we're *too good, and I'm sick of always being sensible.*

Right now, as Lawrence kisses me, Dad's perspective is speaking louder to me than Ingrid's love-bomb warning. Because, okay – maybe I haven't fully let my guard down with Lawrence yet. But does that mean we don't have something great, something worth fighting for?

36.

Rachel

October 2003

And then.

A couple of months later, everything changes.

For about a fortnight – or maybe longer – my body has known. I have felt vaguely unwell, tired in a wired kind of way. Coffee has begun tasting off, as if the milk in it is sour, though Lawrence disagrees. I've started sleeping through my alarm, feeling faintly queasy while brushing my teeth.

It must have happened the night Lawrence and I made it up at the office, back in August. A friend of his had called while we were finishing the wine, to say he had a table at the opening of a new club in town. We were feeling good, already giddy on the drug of reconciliation. So we called a taxi and went to join him.

Things got messy, that night. So messy, I can barely recall most of it.

I do remember the make-up sex, though, when we got back to Lawrence's flat. Frantically cathartic, up against his kitchen counter, both of us high on adrenaline and pent-up lust, the rush of reconnection.

The next morning, I was so hungover, I threw up and had to call in sick. I spent most of the following two days in bed, and messed up my pill timings entirely.

* * *

We have been dating less than a year. But, when I look in the bathroom mirror after taking the test, I feel a flare of happiness so powerful, I have to grip on to the sink with both hands.

I am going to be a mum.

It is a cyclone of a feeling. Thrilling, and electric, and terrifying.

I don't think about Josh. I refuse to let him even enter my mind.

Having called in sick again this morning, I end up pacing my flat for the rest of the afternoon. It is a primal response, I think, to the excitement and fear barrelling through me, and – crazily, already – love.

I have to keep checking the pregnancy test, as if the lines might somehow have reverted to a blank window since I took it.

I want to call Polly, and Ingrid, and my dad. But I can't risk any of them muddying this decision for me. I can't even allow Lawrence to do that.

I cannot tell him. Not until I am sure.

I fire up Yahoo, search for stories of people who became pregnant very early in their relationships. I pore over accounts of couples who, decades later and five kids down, are still happy. Slowly, incrementally, certainty begins to shore up inside me. Why shouldn't it work out that way for us? If being with Josh taught me anything, it's that the life you plan is often a universe away from the one you end up living.

Anyway, things have been going better lately, with Lawrence. We've told our colleagues we're dating now. And he recently surprised me with a weekend trip to Bath, after overhearing me telling Polly I'd never been. I'm making an effort, as well, to resist thinking too far into the future, or constantly revisiting the past.

Somehow, our relationship has begun to feel lighter, and yet deeper.

I even introduced him to Dad over lunch last month. It went well, I think, though the occasion felt a touch too formal, the conversation sometimes stilted. I'd suggested pints at the pub, but Lawrence talked me into four courses at a smart fish restaurant. I know that was only because he was so keen on impressing my dad, though.

Anyway. I'm trying not to worry too much about what Dad thinks. Because, as Lola has wisely reminded me, Dad loved Josh, and look how that worked out. Maybe the precipice of parenthood is the point at which you need to start listening to your own instincts over anyone else's. Perhaps this is just another situation where I need to shut my eyes, trust my gut and take a leap.

I ask Lawrence to drop by my flat after work. I wait for him on the sofa with a knocking heart, the positive test in my hand.

A little after seven, I hear him clatter through the front door, swearing loudly.

Trepidation skates through me. 'What's up?'

He appears in the doorway, water dripping from his hair and coat and face. 'Pissing it down,' he says breathlessly.

I glance towards the window. He's right. Long tails of grey rain are sweeping sideways against the glass, but I hadn't even noticed.

He vanishes into the bedroom while I remain where I am, beginning to doubt my timing.

Eventually, he re-emerges, in jeans and a fresh shirt, rubbing his hair with a towel. He comes over to kiss me without noticing what I am holding.

'You look handsome damp,' I say, because it is true.

'Must try to get caught in more downpours, then.' He flops on to the sofa and discards the towel, stifling a yawn. 'How are you? Feeling better?'

I take a moment to observe him. Maybe I'm being over-cautious: he does seem to be in a good mood, despite the dramatic entrance.

I draw a breath and decide to go for it, passing him the positive test.

He stares at it for a couple of seconds, then looks up at me. 'What the hell? This is amazing.'

'You're happy?'

Dropping the stick, he leans over and pulls me into him, wraps me tightly in his arms. I breathe in the scent of CK One and autumn rain.

'Of course,' he murmurs, voice cracking slightly. 'What did you think I would say?'

'I don't know. It's quick.'

Lawrence has told me several times that he's looking forward to being a dad one day. But that is different from saying, *I would like to have a baby with you.*

He takes my face between his hands, kissing me hard, the way he usually does on a Friday night, or whenever the company share price has spiked. 'I told you from the start I wanted kids.'

'But it's fast. Do you think we can do this?'

He levels his green gaze to mine. Flecks of rainwater still cling to his lashes. Or are they tears? 'Do I reckon we can have a baby? Yeah, Rach, I reckon we can have a baby.'

37.

Josh

October 2003

Somebody's on to me.

The first time, I brush it off as a misdialled number. But the following night it happens again. And then again, the night after that: a phone call that makes me lurch out of bed at two a.m. At the other end of the line, a sinister silence, then the click of the handset being replaced, followed by a dial tone.

And when I'm driving, too, I've begun to get the feeling I'm being followed. A cold-breeze sensation skating over my skin. I keep scanning the rear-view mirror, but it's impossible to tell, of course, if someone is actively tailing you, or if they just happen to be committing the unremarkable offence of driving on the same side of the road.

One night, though, after hanging up on yet another silent phone call, some embedded instinct prompts me to look out of the living-room window. I see a car idling directly opposite my flat, headlights dipped low. Whoever it is drives away as soon as I crank the blinds, the angle and darkness such that I can't see a number plate, or even the make of the car.

I consider going to the police. But what will I say, when they ask who I think it might be? A rogue chemist? A stalker contracted by Big Pharma? I've no doubt the police would be pretty underwhelmed to hear that I think someone might be trying to scare me, no crime's been committed, and no one's been hurt.

I am worried about Wilf, though. If someone out there is prepared to try to intimidate me, I'm pretty sure they'll stop at nothing to get to the man with the million-pound IP. I suspect this is why Wilf has been lying low: he's stopped answering my calls, and, every time I drop by his flat, all the lights are off. It's the longest he and I have gone without speaking in twenty-six years, and I'm struggling to feel okay about it. I even end up calling his mum, who is both surprised to hear from me and slightly confused to have to confirm her only son is still living and breathing.

Talking to her, though, has reminded me of something else. That there is another person I need to speak to, with whom a frank conversation is more than overdue.

Rachel's dad lets me into his house with a guarded smile, as if he's trying to resist saying something slightly sardonic. It would be fair if he did, as he and I haven't spoken in more than two years, since Rachel and I broke up. And, for the entirety of that time, the least I have owed him has been the courtesy of an explanation.

Romantic relationships are so uniquely baffling, in that sense. One day you're as close as it's possible to be, not only with the person you love but the people they love, too. Then, the next, you mess up, and they simply vanish without trace from your life. Not so different from a death. A loss so easily overlooked, but which is a kind of grief, I think.

Rachel's dad makes us tea, then we sit together in the brown cocoon of his seventies-style living room, just as we always did. He even hands me a Tunnock's Teacake, Rachel's number one snack of choice since the day we met. I stare down at it in my hand, the red and silver foil wrapping so familiar, and the sensation of going back in time – and not only aesthetically – hits me harder than I'd been expecting. Because Rachel should be here too, making jokes as she stokes the fire, or telling her dad off about all the out-of-date condiments in his fridge. The three of us should be flipping through old photo albums, or re-watching our wedding video. Rachel should be turning to me in the porch before we let ourselves out, her warm palm to my face as she leans in to kiss me.

Rachel's dad seems to be waiting for me to speak. But my voice is backing up in my throat, the words I'd prepared held back by a dam of unexpressed emotion.

Eventually, I manage to say, 'I owe you an apology. And I have for a long time. I'm sorry for what I did. For how much it must have hurt you, as well as Rachel.'

He nods slowly, sips his tea. 'Thank you, Josh. That means a lot.'

'I should have come to see you sooner. I know that. But I felt . . . too ashamed.'

He seems to consider this. 'Well, you know what they say about shame. It's the only truly useless emotion. Futile. Just holds you back.'

'Maybe,' I say doubtfully, unsure if this lets me off the hook somewhat.

'It stopped you coming to see me, didn't it?' From across the room, his expression is that of tender reproach. 'Anyway. What's done is done. You'll just have to move on with your life now.'

I'd love to, I think. *But without your daughter, I honestly don't know how.*

'So, you believe the pill has worked?'

'It's too early to tell, probably.'

'Well, you look just the same as the last time I saw you. No wrinkles yet.' He winks at me, because his own face, of course, is full of them.

I clear my throat, because there is more I need to say. 'You should know . . . I didn't want to betray her. That was never my intention. I panicked, that night. I just ... didn't think it was possible I'd be the first one in my family to make it past thirty. The chances seemed *so* low.'

'And how do you feel now that a little time has passed?'

It's a chasm of a question, against which all potential responses seem as meagre as specks of dust.

'I wish things could have been different.'

He smiles at me for a long moment, as if he still thinks fondly of me, even now. 'I think we all wish that.'

My breath hitches. Has Rachel said as much? Or is her dad not a fan of Lawrence? Is he trying to find a way to bring Lawrence into the conversation? Or does he want me to?

'Still. There's no changing what's happened,' he continues, before I can say anything. 'And, unkind as this might sound, I think Rachel made the right decision, leaving. I think a future for you two now would be more or less impossible.'

I swallow hard. Because, while this is true, it's always going to sting, hearing your father-in-law say – if we boil it down – that he's glad his daughter gave you the boot.

Still. It's no more than I deserve. 'You're not being unkind. You're being entirely fair.'

He gazes at me and shakes his head, a rare expression of disappointment from the most easy-going guy I've ever known. 'What a waste, Josh. Honestly.'

Alarmingly – because I don't want to cry in front of him – I feel heat shoot to my eyes. 'I know. I'm sorry.'

'You had your whole damn lives ahead of you.'

'I know that too.'

38.

Rachel

November 2003

'Bloody *hell*,' Ingrid says, when I finally share my news with her and Poll.

Polly pulls me into her arms and squeezes so tightly, I panic momentarily that she might squash the bump.

'Have to say I'm relieved. I thought you'd lost your tiny mind, walking into a pub and ordering Ribena.' Ingrid raises her wine glass. 'Anyway. Right. A toast to you both.'

I'm not sure if she means me and Lawrence, or me and the baby. But we all cheers anyway.

'We're thrilled for you, Rach,' Polly says.

'Really?'

Her smile slips slightly. 'Of course. What did you think we would say?'

'I wasn't sure. You're not exactly Lawrence superfans.'

Polly looks worried. 'Rach, Lawrence is honestly very—'

'That's because no one, my darling, could ever be good enough for you,' Ingrid interjects firmly, saving Polly from the perilous task of having to list what she likes about Lawrence.

I smile at Ingrid, shake my head. 'Yeah, yeah.'

'Is he excited?' Polly asks.

I tell her yes, and it isn't a lie. Last night, Lawrence came home with a musical baby mobile hung with tiny felt moons, and a pair of yellow curtains covered in bunnies for the nursery. He'd picked up a Mothercare brochure too, and we spent a soothing couple of hours curled up on the sofa together, going over all the things we might need. Last week he gave me a gift-wrapped book of baby names, surprising me further with the shortlist he'd been working on.

These small demonstrations of commitment have been blindsiding in the best way. Lawrence, as it turns out, is not a love-bomber after all.

I notice Polly kick Ingrid beneath the table, and realise Ingrid is probably itching to ask if I'm sure, to check I have no doubts. Because that is the kind of friend she is.

But it's clear she and Polly have already argued about this, and that – by some miracle – Polly has won. So instead, Ingrid just asks me the question without words.

'I'm really happy,' I assure them both softly.

'We can tell,' Polly says, smiling till the edges of her eyes give way.

'So, when are you going to break the news to Josh?' Ingrid asks.

I know I should be the one to tell him. He deserves to hear it from me. But I'm not too sure how I would even begin to find the words. Words I know will say far too much – and yet, at the same time, nowhere near enough.

39.

Josh

December 2003

One night close to Christmas, I get home from teaching to discover the communal front door to my flat is wide open.

I glance around, expecting to see my upstairs neighbour emptying her bins, or fussing again about the buddleia growing through our gutters. But she is nowhere to be seen.

In the hallway, something feels off. I sense it instantly: atoms, shifting. The tangible, still-warm silence of someone having left in a hurry.

My flat door is open, too.

Inside, everything has been turned over. Drawers upside down, their contents leaking everywhere. Cushions flung from the sofa. The rug a crumple on the floor. Every picture frame dismantled.

I walk gingerly through the flat. Each room is the same: not a single item is where I left it. In the living room, some of the floorboards have even been jemmied up.

I know instantly what they were looking for.

More pills.

Fuck.

I head urgently into the bedroom, squat in front of the fireplace. I feel behind the surround, where my fingers make contact with a little plastic bag, the hard edges of a pill inside it. My shoulders sink with relief.

I decide to leave it in situ, since whoever it is that frisked my flat clearly ruled out this spot as a potential hiding place. So I'm pretty sure that, for now, it's safe.

I get to my feet and shut all the doors. Then I call Wilf, and Rachel. I have to warn them.

The person responsible for this clearly believes – incorrectly – that there's a spare stash of pills somewhere. And if they know I was living with Rachel at the time this all went down, it wouldn't be a huge leap for them to conclude she might have some too.

Neither Wilf nor Rach picks up. So I decide to go to them.

Rachel lives closer, so I head there first. I haven't yet been to her flat, in the two and a half years since she moved out. I've not even felt the urge to drive over there – those fleeting couple of minutes on Valentine's night aside – since the reality of her new life is not an image I've been particularly keen to cement in my mind.

Her building smells brand new, and overwhelmingly of carpet cleaner. The lights are mortuary-bright. It feels the opposite of homely. More like an office block, or the kind of place they send you to sit your driving theory test.

I knock on Rachel's wood-effect door and wait, heart pounding. But it is not Rachel who opens it.

Lawrence wipes his hands on a tea towel, shirt sleeves rolled up to his elbows. He is wearing one of those irritating Statue of David aprons that was doing the rounds as a prank gift a couple of years back.

Dark hair, and unnaturally tanned for the middle of December. Eyes so green they look almost reptilian. From his wrist glints a giant metal man-bracelet, and I find myself wondering if Rachel gave it to him.

For reasons I will never understand, people are always

saying that Lawrence and I look alike. Yes, from a distance, maybe, or if you'd been doing shots. But, up close, he's far more blunt-featured than me, and overly preened. It's ironic that he works in finance, since he is exactly how I would imagine a Ponzi scheme salesman to look.

I admit I am slightly envious of his gleaming jawline, though. After I took the pill, Wilf reminded me that if I shaved (I was due, at the time), my stubble would never grow back. So now, for me, it's between looking permanently as if I'm either en route to a job interview, or crawling out of a tent after four nights at Glastonbury.

Lawrence fake-hesitates, the ghost of a smile crossing his face. 'Josh, right?'

Nodding, I lie through my teeth. 'Good to meet you.'

He takes the hand I've offered him, then shakes it so firmly he practically shatters the metacarpals.

From behind him drifts a smell I recognise well: frying chicken, garlic and tarragon. The scent of one of Rachel's favourite dinners, when we were together. We got it from a Naked Chef recipe I pulled out of a magazine, and I cooked it so often I think even now I could probably remember how.

'I need to talk to Rach. It's pretty urgent.'

'I'll tell her you dropped by,' he says, in a voice that suggests the opposite. He starts to close the door, but I stick out a foot.

'Please. I wouldn't ask if it wasn't important.'

'I really don't want anything stressing her out right now, Josh.'

I hesitate. 'Why? Is she okay?'

The smile returns, only this time it is slightly more triumphant. 'Yeah, she's great, actually. Sorry – didn't you know? She's four months pregnant. We're expecting a baby.'

For a moment, I physically cannot speak. A hot wash of shock begins to ulcerate its way through my stomach lining.

That was fast, is what I'd say if I could. Although, *fast* is actually an understatement. *The most unlike Rachel thing she's ever done* would be more accurate.

Because the truth is, I know Lawrence. He is one of those people who has what I've always thought of as a riptide personality. An invisible undercurrent, far too easy to misjudge.

The exact opposite, in other words, of the person Rachel is.

But if I ever needed evidence that she has moved on for good, I guess now I have it.

And this, ultimately, is why she left. I know that. So that she could have a future – an entirely normal future – with someone she loves.

'Congratulations,' I manage, though my voice sounds a bit like I've cracked a rib.

'Thanks,' Lawrence replies, then waits, his expression a punchable combination of dismissive and smug.

He is trying to goad me, I realise, with his smirk and self-satisfied stance.

And he very nearly succeeds. It takes everything I have – *everything* – to contain myself. But I have already dabbled in being the kind of guy who can't control his emotions, and it's never as gratifying as I want it to be.

I try to focus, and say what I came here to say, warn him about the burglary. In the end, though, it is too hard, like attempting to be coherent after being run over. So I leave without saying another word.

I drive to Wilf's place, thoughts zip lining through my head the whole way.

Rachel is pregnant. Rachel is pregnant.

I can't stop picturing it. Rachel with a bump. The two of them making plans. Decorating a nursery. Buying toys, and books, and sleepsuits. Finding out the sex. Picking names. The hospital bag. The flutters of excitement. The damn *journey* of it all. Everything we dreamed of, talked about, made plans for, for so long.

When I get to Wilf's flat, I'm prepared to see the whole place swathed in darkness, as it usually is. But tonight, instead, I see something else that makes my stomach turn over.

A sign outside. *To Let*.

40.

Rachel

May 2004

I have been sketching my way through pregnancy, creating a time capsule of snapshots I can look back on in years to come. Lawrence's hand on my belly, the first time I felt the baby kick. The cucumbers I couldn't stop eating whole, as though they were apples. Lawrence assembling the cot. The view from our newly decorated nursery window at night, a felt-moon mobile suspended in the foreground. And Lawrence, captured one evening after coming home from the office, feet up, so absorbed in a baby book he didn't even notice me get my sketchbook out.

But later that night, when I looked back at the picture, I was horrified to realise I had drawn Josh in Lawrence's place. It was Josh engrossed in the baby book with his feet up. Josh who was so excited to become a dad, he was reading up on what to expect at every chance he got.

I ripped the picture into tiny pieces and squashed them deep, deep down into the kitchen bin. And then I stood and stared at the closed lid, my body stiff with shock.

Emma Lily Carmichael surprises everyone by making her entrance into the world on a bright Wednesday in May, two weeks ahead of schedule.

Lawrence – unlike his daughter – is late.

Still Falling For You

He headed out this morning for a full day of meetings, his mobile phone switched to silent. As soon as the contractions kicked in I left messages at the office, but these seemed to be interpreted merely as updates, no action necessary. He finally became reachable mid-afternoon, by which point I was incapable of forming full sentences and Polly had to do the bulk of the yelling at him, informing him the baby was nearly here and to get his arse down to the hospital immediately.

Just before he arrives – as I am midway through the long helter-skelter of pain and euphoria and exertion – I get out my phone and begin to text Josh, before Polly takes it gently from my hand, whispering, 'No, sweetie.'

I don't even know why I wanted to contact him, really. A primal urge perhaps, rising up inside me now along with all the others. Or perhaps I still feel guilty, that Lawrence was the one to tell Josh about the baby. My last text to him was an apology, because he hadn't heard it from me.

But then comes another contraction, so the message to Josh remains unsent. Which is probably a good thing, since he might have replied, and this is the point at which Lawrence finally clatters through the door, swearing and complaining about the traffic. He asks the midwives if there are any free plug sockets for him to charge his phone, then informs them he has a mild phobia of hospitals and already feels a little faint. But I just have to leave him to Polly, as the waves of noise and pain and pressure close over my head, pulling me into a place where I am utterly alone, with only one precious purpose.

And now, she has arrived, and it is so surreal, to feel her tiny weight in my arms at last. Finally meeting her, my unblinking gaze latched to hers, after endless nights of reading to her, and sketching the shape of her in my stomach, and talking her through the plot intricacies of the latest series of *24*. I felt I'd got to know her; but this is something else entirely. My love feels boundlessly, extraordinarily vast. Already too big for my arms, this room, the world. A universe all of its own.

Polly has gone home to get some sleep, and Lawrence has nipped out for food, to update his parents and the rest of our friends, and probably check his email.

The room, temporarily, is empty. But I am not alone. I can hear nothing now but our two hearts, beating.

She is already, without a doubt, the best risk I ever took.

I dip my head to hers, which is thick with hair, drawing in the warm, milky smell of her. 'I promise,' I whisper, 'I will be the best mother I can be to you. Always.'

I cannot stop looking into the tiny dark galaxies of her eyes. Right now, I only need her.

My daughter, after so many years of waiting, is finally here.

41.

Rachel

July 2004

Laughably, Lawrence and I came up with what we'd thought to be a fairly watertight plan, for after Emma arrived. We agreed to stay together five nights out of seven, leaving two nights flexible in case of travel, or work meetings, or really terrible sleep.

But it takes Lawrence all of three weeks to begin heading back to his place most nights, so he can – in his words – stand half of a chance of not turning up at work looking as if he's slept in a bus depot.

His daytime calls and messages have become increasingly sporadic, the excuses ramping up. He starts saying, late afternoon most Fridays, that there's been some kind of data- or compliance-related cock-up at the office, which means he has to work all weekend so as not to upset the ombudsman.

We have frequent arguments. Some of them trivial, some not so.

Like one Saturday, as I am sitting in the armchair with Emma and we are disagreeing – again – over why he has to leave so often. The table next to me, much like the rest of my flat, is a sea of snacks and half-drunk cups of tea and paracetamol packets and nipple balm and muslins.

'What if it's damaging Emma? All this coming and going.'

Lawrence laughs derisively, rubs his face. 'She's two months old, Rachel.'

On the back of my neck, sweat prickles. 'Attachment is really important during the early—'

'Actually, babies under six months don't have a preference for any particular adult, as long as they're being well cared for.' He spins this little factoid at me with a note of triumph, as if he's been saving it up for precisely this moment.

Blinking back tears, I think of my mother. I've been starting to wonder lately if I have somehow inherited her dysfunction. Are Lawrence and I destined to be defective too? I try not to fixate on this, but the worry only gets worse the more tired I get.

'Lawrence, that's really—'

'You signed up for this. You knew the deal. We both did.'

'What deal?'

'That we were having a baby before we'd lived together. That we were still just having fun. If you wanted to be married with a joint bank account and picket fence before we did this, then *we should have bloody waited.*'

I stare at him, open-mouthed. 'How can you possibly say that to me while I'm holding our daughter?'

But he just turns his back, as if my question is rhetorical.

I feel hot and sweaty and exhausted. I am craving a shower, to sleep, to tame my tangled hair, to brush the taste of biscuit from my mouth. But what I am desperate for, more than anything else, is a hug.

For some reason – delirium, probably – Aruba floats into my mind. The holiday Josh wanted to take us on, three years ago. The kind of indulgence I've never experienced in my life. I fantasise about it sometimes. Diving into a warm blue sea. Sleeping spreadeagled in bed for as long as I want. Ingesting, at the very least, food that contains some vitamins.

I realise my worst fears are coming true. That having a baby is threatening to crush Lawrence and me, the shape of our future collapsing fast, like clay spinning out of control on a potter's wheel.

Is this how it was for my parents?

I haven't dared to ask Dad yet, not in so many words. Because I think a big part of me would rather not know. Denial to me right now is survival. Sometimes, it is all that carries me through the days.

Lawrence leaves because he can, because he does not have a newborn attached to his body. He slams the door with such force it makes a hairline crack in the wall, and Emma cries so hard, I feel guilt like I've never known.

42.

Josh

August 2004

At the pub, Giles says, 'By the way, I've heard it's not all roses between Rachel and her man. Lo says they're fighting. Like, a lot.'

I stare at him. 'What do you mean, fighting?'

'Nothing physical. Just ... they row. Quite badly, Lo reckons.'

I know arguing's pretty common when you've just had a baby. But still, I'm concerned. Rachel and I would fall out from time to time, like any couple. Yet I'd have struggled to describe any of those disagreements as fights.

Later, I send her a message. Because I need to know.

Part of me expects radio silence. Mere minutes later, though, she calls.

It is the first time we have spoken since she had the baby.

'Congratulations,' I say softly, though it comes out slightly falsetto, because my mouth is so dry.

There is a long silence. So long, in fact, that I begin to wonder if she has butt-dialled me by accident.

I am sitting topless on the edge of my bed, a fan grinding away because it's so damn hot. Even now this room still feels like ours, filled as it is with little hints of the life we once shared. The duvet cover we picked out. The chest of drawers we butchered together without looking at the instructions, stripping every single screwhead as we went. The curtain pole we put up with no spirit level, so there's always a gap when they're drawn.

Eventually, Rachel speaks. 'Thank you for your card. It was lovely.'

'Sorry I haven't called before now. But I thought it best to . . . you know.'

'I know.'

I last saw her at Easter, in a beer garden a few weeks before Emma was born. She looked radiantly happy. At one point, Lawrence put his hand on her belly and made eye contact with me at exactly the same time, which felt childish at best, creepy at worst. I left pretty soon after that, to deprive him of the rise it was clear he was seeking.

'How's everything going? How's Emma?' My voice keels a little as I say her name.

'She's perfect,' she whispers. She is eating something. I don't ask what, though my money's on a Tunnock's Teacake.

I might as well be straight with her. 'Lola said—'

'That was just a stupid row about . . . God, I can't even remember. Formula, or something.' She sighs heavily, as if this isn't the first time she's had to defend Lawrence.

'But serious enough for you to tell Lola?'

'She caught me at a bad moment. Lo and Polly and Ingrid . . . they're not exactly the I-heart-Lawrence fan club. I assume you've heard.'

I hadn't, actually. Though I'm hardly surprised. Temperamentally speaking, from what I can work out, the man is the equivalent of dropping a hairdryer in a bath.

For some reason I want to ask if the baby was planned. But I don't, because I know it is none of my business.

I stare blankly for a moment through the gap in the curtains, at the star-strewn night sky.

'I think everyone thinks ...' Rachel begins, then stops herself.

The seconds stretch.

Eventually, she says, 'That Lawrence has a temper, or something. But he doesn't. Not like that, anyway.'

'Okay,' I say slowly. 'So what kind of temper does he have?'

'Please don't,' she mutters. 'You're worse than Polly.'

We lapse into a strained silence. I look down at my hands, my wrist, the watch she gave me that I wear every day.

'You'd tell me,' I say eventually.

I hear her hesitate. 'Hardly fair to make you my relationship counsellor, Josh.'

'Oh, fuck that.'

'Yes,' she concedes. 'I would tell you.'

I take a second to picture her as we talk, sitting in a flat I have never set foot in. I imagine somewhere stylish and calm, brightened now by baby things. Is she wearing his T-shirt? Perfume, or jewellery, he has given her? How long is her hair now? My desperation for detail is at once compulsive and depressing. Not dissimilar to drinking too many pints at the pub, then needing to chuck it all up in a hedge on the way home.

'Are you still sketching?' The question feels important, somehow. Like resting two fingers against her wrist, gently taking her pulse.

'When I have time.' I hear her swallow. 'I do miss you, Josh. I wish we could talk more.'

I feel sadness whorl through me as she says this. Sparks of anguish, just spinning, with nowhere to go. 'Can't really help you there,' I say softly.

She lets out a breath. 'I know. Sorry. That was ... I'd better go.'

'Rachel?'

'Yeah.'

Still Falling For You

'Promise me something.'

'Okay.'

'I'll always be here for you.'

A few moments pass, and I realise I've misworded it.

'I mean, just . . . pick up the phone. If you ever need to. It doesn't matter if it's three o'clock in the morning. I'm here, okay?'

She doesn't say anything else, just gently ends the call. But I can tell from the way she is breathing that she is trying not to cry.

43.

Rachel

September 2004

Today is Tuesday, I think. Lawrence stayed over last night, but ended up vanishing into the spare bedroom in the early hours. I felt him ease out of bed, tiptoe to the door. But I was already awake, lost in the darkened room as if it was outer space. Floating, alone, connected to nothing.

We have sat mostly in silence on the sofa since he got up, while he's replied to emails and downed a couple of espressos. He installed a posh coffee machine here a few weeks back. It takes up as much space as a small car on the worktop in my kitchen.

He gets to his feet now, moves over to the sink. 'For God's sake,' he mutters, trying to squeeze his cup in among the mound of dirty dishes. 'This flat looks like a fucking squat.'

He is freshly showered, his work clothes clean, his cologne crisp. He smells to me of a past life I feel guilty for missing, sometimes. He has time for everything – to have breakfast and caffeinate, to wash and shave and linger in front of the mirror, to spend more than a millisecond picking out his clothes.

I look down at our baby, feeling my heart swell at the sight of her in her little koala-print sleepsuit, a gift from Lola and Giles.

'Can you clean up a bit today?' Lawrence says. He goes to stand in front of the mirror by the door, pushing a hand through his hair before carefully peeling a whitening strip from his teeth. He discards it and smacks his lips, pats an eyebrow into place with a fingertip. 'It can't make you feel very good, living in squalor.'

I stare at him for a long time, trying wildly to remember all my reasons for having wanted to be with him in the first place. For desiring him enough that nothing else mattered. And missing Josh so heavily that every other choice seemed somehow weightless.

He catches my eye in the mirror. 'Tell me I'm wrong.'

Okay, I think. *Okay, then, I will tell you.* 'Well, she feeds every ninety minutes, Lawrence, I'm doing ten nappy changes a day, she hates being put down, I'm so tired I'm genuinely worried I could fall asleep and crush her to death, I can't remember the last time I ate a vegetable and my body hasn't felt like my own for I don't know how long. But sure. Let's talk about the dirty dishes.'

'And yet you still have time to draw.' He picks up my sketchbook as though it's evidence of a crime. 'You have time to do this.'

'Yes. For ten minutes here and there, because it helps me to feel half-human.'

'Call me crazy,' he says, 'but I think it might benefit our daughter – and you – if you used that time more productively.'

'Well, thanks, I'm in desperate need of tips on productivity *and* parenting right now, Lawrence.'

But I know the anger I am feeling is not actually directed at Lawrence. It is at myself, for knowing things would turn out this way – because I *did* know – and choosing to ignore it.

He holds up his hands, as if he is the one being attacked. 'I'm just saying. It's been four months. I thought we'd be back to some sort of normality by this point. Christ, you don't even let me touch you.'

Until now, I've been eager to assure everyone that Lawrence is a good father, perhaps because he is the kind of guy who naturally inspires doubt. And it hasn't felt like a lie: he does change nappies and take the baby as soon as he's home, winding her and playing with her and bathing her, even driving her round the block at midnight in his car to get her to settle. He does try, with Emma.

But he no longer tries with me.

And being a good father, I am starting to realise, is not only about the baby.

'You know I'm still in pain,' I say, my emotions like steam inside me, building, building. 'Why would you—'

'Don't twist my words. It's not just about that.'

'I think it is,' I say, because the truth is, I know Lawrence. I always have. But I wouldn't admit it, because I couldn't face up to what being attracted to him meant about me.

He looks at me for a long time. The skin above his collar has turned red. 'It's fine if you don't want me, Rachel. Whatever. But the truth is, I don't want you either, when you're like this.'

'*When I'm like this*. A new mother, trying to keep our daughter alive.'

I see the exact moment at which his temper ignites. I know it so well, I could almost count it down. The flaming skin. The sudden charge to his eyes. The flattened lips and rigid jaw. 'Don't be so fucking dramatic. Millions do it, every day. You need to *get it together*, Rachel.'

Suddenly, the warm weight of my daughter in my arms feels like everything on earth I want to fight for. Sanity and wellbeing, happiness, calm.

I think back to what I whispered to her in the hospital, when she was mere minutes old. *I promise I will be the best mother I can be to you. Always.*

And my heart is remembering, too, what my father once told me. *Sometimes, staying means holding out for changes that will never come. Accepting something that is irretrievably broken, and losing yourself in the process.*

'Lawrence . . . I think you should leave.'

'Don't worry, I am.' He grabs his car keys. 'I'm already late.'

'No.'

The room falls silent, the space between us changing colour, getting darker and yet lighter as I finally say what needs to be said.

'I mean, *leave*. This isn't working.'

Lawrence shows no emotion – no sadness or surprise, nothing resembling regret. Instead, he clears his throat, scratches a spot of skin just below his ear, and says, 'Well, I guess one of us had to say it. I've been thinking the same thing. For weeks, actually.'

'Okay.' I allow him this final ego prop, because what does it matter, now?

He jabs a finger in my direction. 'You know you have serious attachment issues? You're going to end up dying alone.'

I shut my eyes as I wait for the father of my baby to leave my flat and not come back.

SECTION III

44.

Rachel

March 2005

I've been sketching and painting every day, in the six months since Lawrence and I broke up. I draw while Emma feeds and sleeps, one-handed if I need to, while I could be washing, or napping, or getting my fix of trash TV. I trawl artists' websites, hungry for inspiration. I see art in everything – the slant of light on a building, the texture of water creased by wind, a perfectly angled streetscape. I dream of pigments and patterns, colours colliding on canvases.

So, eventually, I decide to hand in my notice at the bank, before my maternity leave is up, to try to make a go of my art. My plan is to start slowly, accepting commissions for friends and acquaintances, and see where it takes me. Josh was always encouraging me to do this, when we were together. But I never felt brave enough. Now, though, feels like the right time to take the leap. And as Polly pointed out the other night, 'If you don't do it now, you never will.'

Lawrence, of course, thinks it's a terrible idea. He says I'll barely scrape by, that his mother – a semi-famous artist – makes a pittance. He insists I'll never get another job as good as the one I already have, one that comes with annual leave and pension contributions and big fat bonuses.

And there is truth to some of that. But there is another truth inside me too, one I feel far more acutely. Which is that it's time for a fresh start. I *need* a fresh start. In years to come, I want Emma to look at me and be proud of the person I am.

To my immense relief, it didn't take Lawrence and me long to establish a tentative truce after we parted ways. It became apparent fairly quickly that we work far better apart than we ever did together. And, right now, nothing is more important to me than making sure his bond with his daughter remains tight. No matter what's gone on between us, as long as I have breath in my body I will fight for Emma to know and love her father.

After Lawrence drops Emma home one Sunday night in March, I make tea and bathe her, then settle her down.

I never thought I'd miss the early days of night feeding, but, weirdly, I do. I remember it – far too nostalgically, of course – as girl time. Just the two of us, bonding as I consumed endless snacks and drinks and hours upon hours of mindless TV.

Once I'm back in the living room, and the flat has fallen quiet, my mind turns – as it so often does – to Josh.

This has been happening more and more frequently lately.

I think of him when I'm in bed, the flat dark and dormant. I find myself imagining him next to me. Touching me. Kissing me. The things he might whisper about what he wants us to do.

We haven't spoken in seven months. Since he said I could always ring him, no matter what the time was.

So, tonight, I take him at his word. I get out my phone, and send him a text.

45.

Josh

March 2005

'Can I see her?'

Rachel smiles and nods, beckons me gently to Emma's room. It is a primrose-hued cocoon, filled with baby rabbits and bunting and gingham, the soft glow of a nightlight.

Together, we go in. I step over to her cot, look down at her sleeping.

She is beautiful, of course. Just like her mum.

The emotions arrive fast and thick, monsooning their way up my throat. I try very hard to focus on the entirely bonkers fact that this tiny human is half Rachel.

'This is mad, Rach. You have a baby. You *made* her.'

It could have been us. It should *have been us.*

Rachel's smile is peaceful and content. Not at all like she's mourning everything we could have been.

She's moved on, I realise. Because of course she bloody has.

I came over to Rachel's place at the speed of light, the moment I received her text. I've composed and junked so many of my own to her in the months since we spoke on the phone. But it's never felt like a good time, or that I have any of the right words. I didn't want to get in the way of her and Lawrence, much as I can't stand the guy. But, since I heard they broke up, the urge to contact her has been stronger than ever.

Darren warned me off. 'You don't want people to think you're swooping in.'

'In what way would I be swooping in?'

He extended one arm into a kind of Superman pose. 'You know.'

I gave him a bemused thumbs-up. 'Right. Thanks. That helps.'

'You get what I'm saying. Just give her some time.' He shrugged. 'Maybe wait until she calls you.'

Now, in the living room, Rachel pours some wine, and we sit down together on the sofa.

She has told our friends before now that she feels permanently haggard since having Emma. But to me, tonight, she looks utterly the opposite. Skin mellow in the lamplight, blonde hair spilling over her shoulders, caramel eyes gleaming. She is wrapped up in a giant sweatshirt, joggers and big socks, because it is still so cold outside.

Her flat is nice, in the sense that everything works, and nothing leaks or creaks. But I wonder if she ever thinks about our old home. Its character features and wonky floors, battered walls, rambling garden.

Probably not. My mind rewinds to the two-up, two-down new build she was so taken with, just before we offered on the flat. Perhaps, in fact, this is the life her heart wanted all along, before I persuaded her it was a better idea for us to buy a place where you wake up every morning wondering what new bit of it has fallen off overnight.

Cautiously, I ask what happened with Lawrence. I've heard the story second-hand, of course. But I'm curious for her version.

She swigs from her glass, shakes her head. It's hard, I guess, to distil the end of what you shared with another person into a sentence or two.

'I was expecting it to be stressful, at times, with a newborn. But we were fighting constantly. For literally no reason.'

I am tempted to suggest that maybe the reason was Lawrence, a man who seems to spreads ill-feeling like it's an STI.

'Am I allowed to tell you what I really think of him yet?'

She nudges me with her foot. 'I already know what you really think.'

'Ah, go on. Please let me.'

'No. I'm rising above it.'

I decide to save calling her ex out on his behavioural gonorrhoea for another day. Because, really, I know it is not my place.

'I'm sorry,' I say, out of nowhere. 'I'm so sorry I fucked everything up, Rachel.'

She doesn't reply. But I see her eyes spring swiftly with tears.

For a moment, neither of us can speak. Then she clears her throat, gets up to fetch us both a refill.

'How are things with you?' she asks, returning after several minutes with more wine and having just checked on Emma. 'Still no sign of Wilf?'

I shake my head. Not long after the *To Let* sign went up outside Wilf's flat, I drove past again to see the board gone and all the lights on. I emergency-braked, jumped out of the car, then hammered on the door. The slightly bemused and bespectacled man inside had no idea where his new landlord was, though he did say he'd got a European ringtone when he tried to call him about the boiler.

It's been nearly two years since Wilf and I last spoke. And I miss him, deeply. I realise now I took him for granted, in the same way you do the birds in the sky. He was always just there. I feel his absence as I would if birdsong were to vanish from the earth forever.

Rachel asks if I'm writing at the moment. I tell her *kind of*, though the truth is, since my fifth novel came out to precisely no acclaim last year I've been experiencing the worst creative block of my life. No ideas for a new one will stick. So I've taken to just doodling nonsense long into the night, drinking whisky from the bottle I keep in the filing cabinet. Watching videos of cats falling into buckets on the internet. Wondering if I should ditch Friends Reunited in favour of Facebook. Repeatedly typing *Wilfred Merryfield* into Google.co.uk.

How long it takes for my thoughts to stray to the choice I made nearly five years ago usually depends on how much whisky I've drunk. But invariably I go there, torturing myself with fantasies of how different things might be, if I'd never taken that pill. Whether Rachel and I would have kids of our own by now. Might we have moved house, found a lovely old wreck in the countryside, perhaps? Got a dog, a couple of cats? Maybe my happiness, in this parallel fantasy life, would even have inspired me to write a book that would sell in its millions.

'You're not going to give up, are you? I read your book, just before I had her.'

Rachel's forehead is so deeply furrowed when she says this, I almost reach for her hand.

It always smarts, catching sight of her bare ring finger. It still feels, on many levels, unbelievable. I've carried on wearing mine. I don't know if that's weird. It probably is.

I shake my head. 'Perhaps I should go away for a while. Maybe Wilf had the right idea, escaping abroad.'

Rachel nods, a faraway look in her eye. 'God, yeah. You know, I still think about Aruba sometimes, when I'm—' She breaks off, and laughs. 'Well, delirious from lack of sleep, essentially.'

It takes everything I have not to tell her to pack a bag. That I'll put a holiday for two – three – to Aruba on my credit card right now.

'Your writer's block probably just needs a muse,' Rachel says.

I half-laugh, because I appreciate irony, and look down at my knees. Since we broke up, I've begun to wonder if Rachel *was* my muse. I haven't told her this, mostly because I don't think she'd enjoy the guilt trip, plus the concept has always seemed faintly patriarchal to me. But still. I can't shake the feeling that, since she left, my brain doesn't work in quite the same way as it did. Is it that I'm unhappy? Or that I can't fully relax?

I got talking to Darren about this not long ago. But all he did was try to persuade me to start smoking a very potent grade of weed.

'Do you have one, at the moment?' she asks. 'A muse.'

'Do you mean, am I seeing anyone?'

She smiles. 'I was trying to be subtle.'

I laugh. 'Okay. But just so you know? Ingrid on an acid trip is more subtle than you.'

The funny thing is, I want to tell her. I like that she wants to know. But what I can't confess is that, a full four years on, I still can't kiss anyone else without thinking of her.

Instead, I just tell her that yes, occasionally, I hook up with girls. Without adding, of course, that I have never been able to replicate what we had. That I end every one of these encounters feeling empty and disconnected. I usually tell whoever it is close to nothing about myself, whereupon we have a brief and mutually unsatisfying shag before going our separate ways.

'And? How is it?' Rachel asks.

I hesitate. Make a sound that is not quite a laugh, look away.

'Sorry. I'm being insensitive.'

Maybe. But, with her, it never truly feels like that. I will always want to talk to her about this stuff. No matter how weird it might seem to other people.

'I was trying to think of a more creative word than crap,' I say.

She sips her wine, steadying her brown eyes against me. 'In what way?'

Heart hopping, I meet her gaze. The seconds stretch.

'I guess it's better when you really know the person,' I say eventually. My mouth, abruptly, has gone dry with want. 'Or, you know . . . love them.'

'How much better?'

I see her breath catch, a tiny jump to her chest.

I picture setting down my glass, leaning forward to kiss her. Teasing my tongue into her mouth. Feeling her touch me. Clothes coming off as time turns to liquid. Taking her to the brink with my fingers, hearing her gasp my name.

'So good, you have the kind of sex you can't stop thinking about. Even years later. You know?'

She nods, fiercely. 'Yeah,' she whispers.

And now I do put down my glass, and am about to lean in when a tiny whimper fills the air.

The spell is broken. Rachel turns her head. Emma's cry ramps up.

'Sorry,' Rachel murmurs, setting down her own glass and getting to her feet.

46.

Rachel

March 2005

In Emma's room, once I've settled her, I pause inside her door and draw a few juddering breaths.

I allow myself – just for a moment – to picture it. The first kiss. Leading him to my bed, the place where I have so often thought of him. Peeling the clothes from his body, the things we might whisper to each other. Running my hands across the perfect ridges of his torso. The flex of his muscles, the heat of him inside me.

In a strange way, imagining him like this reminds me of the unreal weeks just before we broke up, when I think we both – even Josh – knew we could not last. I remember how desperately we would reach for each other after dark. The messy heat of craving him, everything sharp and heightened and adrenaline-fed. Like the moments before a parachute jump, pleasure that felt reckless. What strange human impulse makes us do that?

But then would come the confusion, swamping me every morning as I showered the night from my skin.

No. There was a reason you left. This won't solve anything.

Watching him with Emma earlier was more painful than I'd expected. It was so hard not to picture – even for a second – a life in which she was his.

Sometimes, late at night, I have looked down at her sleeping, her fair hair bright against the mattress, and allowed myself to imagine it. That Josh is not only my husband, but my daughter's father, too. That, right now, he is brushing his teeth in the bathroom, or putting dishes away in the kitchen, and will soon slide into bed beside me, his body warm and tight and loyal.

He sent a card when she was born. A teddy bear in a hot-air balloon, surrounded by peachy clouds. He addressed it to both Lawrence and me. And it made me ache a little inside, to think what it must have taken for him to do that.

When I return to the living room, Josh hasn't moved. But I notice his wine glass is empty.

'Maybe . . . we should call it a night,' I say, perching on the edge of the armchair. For the sake of my own resolve, I can't quite look him in the eye.

He doesn't reply for a couple of moments. Then: 'I've been thinking that maybe the effects of the pill can be reversed.'

Just like that.

'What do you mean?'

'I mean, if it was that easy for Wilf to invent it, maybe it wouldn't be too difficult to create an antidote.'

Now, I do look at him. He is leaning forward, elbows on his knees, just the way he used to when he thought the pill was his silver bullet and he was trying to talk me round.

'I didn't get the impression it was easy for Wilf to invent it. And he said it alters your body on a cellular level. He said there's no changing your mind, once you take it.'

'But that was five years ago. Science moves fast. I can make enquiries—'

'Why, though?'

'Because I still love you.' In the low light of the living room, he holds me in his gaze. 'And I know you still have feelings for me.'

My eyes begin to burn. 'Don't tell me what I feel.'

'All right. You tell me, then. Do you still love me?'

He waits for what must be thirty seconds, but I can't reply. My voice is pinned to the wall of my throat.

'If I could find someone who could—'

'Are you saying you regret taking it? I mean, do you even *want* to reverse the effects?'

Because if you do, I think, *you threw our future away for nothing.*

He doesn't move, or hesitate, or answer my question. 'Please just be honest with me, Rach. If I can find an antidote, could we try again?'

47.

Rachel

July 2006

Dad rings to tell me my mother has died. He wants to know if I wish to go to her funeral.

He asks me out of duty, I think, rather than with any realistic expectation that I will say yes. And I decline, of course. We've not spoken since the eighties. According to her sister – with whom Dad last had contact about a decade ago – she ended up moving to the south coast, and quitting journalism to work in advertising.

Over the years, I have felt, of course, the absence of a maternal ear, that background pulse of unconditional love. But I have not felt the absence of *her* in any meaningful way.

I feel fear blow through me when Dad tells me how she died, though. Not for myself, but for my daughter. For the dark cloud that might now forever be hanging on her horizon.

In the end, I'm not sure what impels me to stand opposite the church a fortnight later, watching the funeral cortège roll in. Perhaps a part of me, even now, wants to try to understand. To gain some eleventh-hour clues as to who she was. One final attempt to make sense of her.

If you couldn't love me, couldn't you at least have cared?

But even that question feels wrong, when I think of my

own daughter, the ferocity of my love for her a fire that could never burn out.

So maybe the more fitting question is, *Why couldn't you love me?*

I recognise none of the tiny group of mourners. I try to guess which – if any – of them are her family, friends, lovers. It's not easy. They all look like strangers. I'm not even sure I could pick out Mum's sister now.

And then, for the first time in more than two decades, I see my mother. Or at least, the coffin she is lying in.

After everyone has filed inside, I remain standing in the dappled shade of a horse chestnut tree, just gazing at the church. I try to imagine what they are saying about her in there. Exactly which of her qualities they are eulogising, the parts of her personality they say they will miss.

I picture her blank eyes. The numbness. The never feeling. The never loving.

I wonder if anybody has mentioned that she was a mother once, too.

After an hour or so, they start spilling out on to the pavement again.

And that is her life over. Just like that.

I watch everyone milling around, dabbing their eyes and hugging each other.

And I try to feel something, because surely it would be normal to muster up some kind of sentiment or flicker of emotion – even if it is only relief, or anger? But I just feel numb.

One by one, the mourners disperse. And then the road falls quiet again, the only sound the silky trill of a blackbird singing a final hymn.

* * *

Later, Lawrence arrives to pick Emma up for the weekend. I don't tell him about my mother, or where I've been today.

As soon as they have left I stare into the mirror that hangs in my hallway. I look blank and pale, in a way that seems ghostly, not quite human.

I need to feel something. Any fucking feeling at all.

Apparently, I have, over the course of a single afternoon, acquired my mother's capacity for utter detachment. And that is not something I can bear for one second longer. So I head for the kitchen, where there is still a bottle of tequila left over from Ingrid's birthday last year.

I need to feel something.

48.

Josh

July 2006

It's late for visitors, or delivery drivers. After ten. But my doorbell goes anyway.

When I open the door, Rachel is standing on the front step, eyes a little glazed.

I can see straight away that she is drunk. And I can't help smiling. Because drunk Rachel is actually one of my all-time favourite Rachels.

She eventually asked me to leave, that night I was at her flat and told her I still loved her. We've exchanged the odd text message since. But we haven't spoken properly in over a year.

'My mum died,' is all she says.

I stare at her, confused. As far as I knew, Rachel's had no contact with her mum for a good couple of decades. Should I tell her I'm sorry? Or is this more of a solemn high-five, let's-bitch-about-her-over-a-tumbler-of-whisky kind of situation?

'That's . . . not what I was expecting you to say.'

She leans against the wall of the porch. 'Can I come in?'

I just open the door.

I change my mind about the whisky when Rachel zigzags along my hallway as if she's figure-skating.

'Let's have a drink,' she says, as we head into the living room.

'Nope. No more units for you. I'll get some water.'

'Hey,' she says, stopping abruptly, 'you decorated.'

'Long story,' I say.

I had the bizarre urge, one night, to paint the living room charcoal-grey, to eradicate the magnolia it had been when Rachel lived here. But as soon as I'd finished I realised I hated it. Half an hour later I was back in Homebase, shelling out another forty quid to make it all neutral again.

I guess Rachel has only surmised the walls have turned from magnolia to pale cream. But I'm pleased, deep down, that she has noticed.

'It looks nice.' She sighs, heavily. 'God, I miss this flat.'

I venture a smile, amused despite the churning in my chest. 'As in, the bricks and mortar?'

She nods earnestly, completely missing my implication. 'Yeah. My place is nice, but it's so bland. It's like living inside a yoghurt pot.'

'You've lost me.'

'You know – all-white. A bit sour. None of my neighbours ever says hello.' She sways a little, sits heavily down on the sofa. She adjusts the straps of her green dress, crosses then re-crosses her bare legs. Her skin is kissed with summer, blonde hair a torrent around her shoulders. 'Do you have any coffee?'

'Is that a serious question?'

She looks up and blinks. 'Why, have you run out?'

She sounds so disappointed, my heart crumbles. 'No, of course not. Coming right up.'

In the kitchen, I make coffee stronger than even I usually take it. Then I return to the living room and sit down next to her on the sofa, switch on a lamp.

'Can't believe you still have these,' she says with a smile, patting the Aztec-print cushion next to her. It's one of four

I've held on to since the early nineties, and is an eyesore, quite frankly. But I am pathologically unable to throw anything away.

Rachel's breath is hot, and laced with booze. We used to call it *dragon breath*: pure ethanol. *Steer clear of open flames, Rach*, I would call out, whenever she went to brush her teeth after a particularly heavy night. At which point she would lob something soft at my head, and almost always miss.

She leans against my shoulder, and within moments begins to drift off. Her breath deepens, slowing against my skin. I don't get up, because I just want to keep feeling it.

After about ten minutes, a car door slams outside and Rachel stirs. With some effort, she blinks her eyes open, then swallows.

'Sorry,' she murmurs, shuffling upright.

'Don't be.' I pass her the coffee. 'It's still warm.'

She smiles, takes a sip. 'Thanks.'

I notice her hands are flecked with paint. I heard from Polly via Darren that she quit her job just before her maternity leave was up, to pursue her art. The news made my heart bright with pride, a planet in the strange black hole of my feelings for her. She always used to play down her talent, but it never passed me by just how good she was. Still, I know how much it must have taken, for her to leave her job.

I think it will always sting, that she no longer shares these life changes with me first. That any updates I get are watered-down, second-hand. That I'm not the one she goes to raise a glass with now.

Gently, I ask how her mother died.

'Officially? Pneumonia. But she had dementia. She got it young, apparently. She wasn't even seventy.'

'I'm sorry,' I say, even though I have felt pretty hostile towards Rachel's mother for most of my adult life. But my sympathies are really for Rachel. For the way I know that information will have made her feel.

'I went and stood outside the church earlier.'

'How come?'

'Um, honestly? I don't know. Closure, maybe.'

'And did you get it?'

She wraps her hands around her cup. She seems to be sobering up a little. 'I'm not actually sure. What does closure feel like?'

I just laugh, and shake my head.

'Hey, you still wear your watch,' she whispers.

I look down at it, turn my wrist gently over. 'Why wouldn't I?'

'And your ring.' She raises her eyes to mine. They are still a little weighty from the alcohol.

She's never brought it up before. I suppose she might have wanted to, and not known how. But I don't reply, because there is not really a sentence on earth that could cover it.

Fortunately, she doesn't press me. 'The funeral reminded me how weird life is. You know: one minute you're drinking tequila. The next, you've got dementia, and then you're in a coffin. And people will cry for a bit, but then the world moves on. Which made me think . . .'

She is holding my gaze. My breath kicks in my chest.

'I mean, take now, for example. I'm thirty-six, and you're twenty-nine. That's not really such a big deal, is it?'

'Rach—'

'So maybe you and I should just spend the next few years . . . not worrying about the future till it comes. *If* it even comes. Life is for living, right?'

It's so strange, to hear Rachel talking like this, saying all the same things I was, five years ago. It's very unlike her. But a lot has changed since we broke up. And that's what funerals do for you, I guess.

Still Falling For You

In the next moment, I feel the press of her palm against my face. Gently turning my head to hers, leaning in to kiss me.

With an almighty effort I push her gently away, get to my feet. 'Rach, we can't. I can't.'

She blinks up at me. 'But you said before—'

'That was before. This is now, and you're ... really drunk.'

'I've had coffee,' she protests, as if this is any sort of legitimate argument. But she says it with such sincerity that I almost laugh.

I look down at her, heart cartwheeling. 'I don't ever want to be something you regret in the morning, Rach.'

She tugs her knees into her chest and rests her chin on them, says nothing.

'Sorry,' she whispers, after a while. 'That was lame of me.'

I sit back down, rock gently into her. *Don't worry about it.*

A few moments pass.

'Rach?' I say.

'Yeah.' In the lamplight, her body looks almost completely gold.

The words are out of my mouth before I've even really thought what it is I want to say. 'You should know ... I still have the second pill.'

Her eyes swim a little, then refocus. 'The second pill,' she repeats.

'I thought you might want it now. Given how your mum died, I mean.'

Her brown eyes dart back and forth across my face, as if she's trying to work out when I started shedding brain cells. 'You said you were going to look for an antidote. To reverse the effects. But now you're offering it to me?'

'That was before ... this stuff with your mum. I thought you might want to take something to prevent it, before it—'

'I should go.' She sets down the coffee and gets to her feet, wobbling a little.

I feel a lurching sensation inside me. Like a car hitting ice, the misjudgement all my own. After the last time, I swore to myself I would never offer her that pill again. But, having heard this about her mum, I couldn't not.

'Please don't. You can stay. Please. Have my room, I'll take the sofa.'

She shakes her head, fishes around for her bag. 'I'm sorry I came here. I shouldn't have.'

My heart clenches, hard. 'Rach, forget I said that. Please. I should never have suggested it. I didn't think.'

But in the time it takes me to shut my eyes and punch out a breath of pure frustration, she is gone.

49.

Rachel

September 2007

I have paid to take a stall at a county fair, exhibiting my artwork. All day, the autumn sky has been mineral-blue, the air clean and clear as a rockpool.

It's gone well, but these shows are mostly for browsers. Exhibitions help to raise my profile, getting my name out there and my card into people's hands, but I rarely come away from them with a pocket full of cash.

I am about to start packing up when a silver-haired man approaches and begins to examine my canvases.

'So,' he says, after a short while, turning to face me. 'Financial services' loss really is the art world's gain. Now there's a sentence I never thought I'd say.'

I frown and smile at the same time, shading my eyes with one hand, trying to get a better look at him. He is tall and olive-skinned, hair smartly cropped, a pair of sunglasses hooked into his collared shirt. He looks slightly incongruous in my part of the field; I imagine him feeling far more at home over in the champagne tent.

He smiles back at me, extends a hand. 'Oliver Danvers.' He smells suave, of cedar and rainfall, and has immaculately white teeth. His hair colour doesn't quite tally with the rest of him, in that I wonder if he went grey at an early age.

His name – or is it his voice? – strikes a chord in my brain, but it's hard to know which one, or why.

As our palms lock, I remember. 'Oliver Danvers Recruitment?'

'That's the one.'

'We used to talk on the phone—' I say, then break off, because the women in my department at the bank would always argue over who got to speak to Oliver Danvers when he called, on account of his melted-molasses voice. We even decided at one point he must have missed his vocation manning phone sex hotlines.

'We did,' Oliver says, his smile expanding, so perhaps he's already aware of the sex hotline thing.

I feel my neck begin to redden slightly. 'I hope I was impeccably polite.'

'Oh, you were. In fact, I distinctly remember you giving me the most courteous *get lost* I've ever received.'

I laugh. 'Sorry. Budgets. You know how it is.'

'Absolutely.' His grey gaze grips me. 'Listen, I've got to head off now, but . . . would you fancy going out for a drink some time?'

We meet the following Friday, at a bar in the middle of town. Oliver says he's had a tip from Danny, his business development guy, about a place that does next-level cocktails. Inside, the initial signs are good: it is one of those intimate, lamplit spaces filled with snug leather booths and velvet armchairs, the décor plush and moody. But when we come to order our drinks, it becomes clear that the broader theme of the bar is essentially . . . well, sex.

The neon wall art, vast gallery of naked-person portraits and exclusively rude cocktail list are all beginning to make sense now. That, and the name of the bar: Sweetlove's.

'Danny just said it was retro,' Oliver says, rubbing his face with one hand, after I've encouraged him to see the funny side. 'He obviously thought this would be the prank of the century. I'm looking forward to Monday.'

I'm amused to notice he has gone slightly pink in the face. 'So, tell me,' I ask, 'how is your Screaming Orgasm?'

He groans. 'Really bloody good. Annoyingly enough. And your—' He breaks off and shakes his head. 'Nope. I can't even say it.'

'My Dirty Banana? Delicious.'

He bark-laughs. 'Oh, God. I am sorry, Rachel. You must think—'

'Not at all.' Beneath the table, I nudge my knee against his. 'I mean, it's an ice-breaker, if nothing else.'

'I don't think we really needed one, but . . . thank God it's you,' he murmurs.

I mention Emma at the earliest opportunity, not only because she is my favourite subject, but because I want to eliminate the possibility of any misunderstandings at the outset.

Oliver listens intently, bright-eyed, as I talk about her. Then he says, 'She sounds wonderful. I adore kids. I'm lucky enough to have two nieces. My sister tells me off for spoiling them rotten, but . . .'

I smile. 'What else are uncles for?'

Every now and then, as we chat, our hands or legs brush and we share a smile, let our gazes linger. It is so different from being out drinking with Lawrence, which always felt a bit high-stakes, as if one of us could easily say the wrong thing or misjudge the moment at any point, whereupon the whole night would instantly darken, the mood turning sour and wrong.

But it doesn't once feel that way with Oliver.

We get another round in. Oliver has relaxed a bit now, orders a Knickerdropper Glory without flinching. I go for a couple of Slippery Nipples, because I haven't done shots in ages.

'You know,' he says at one point, 'whenever I called your office, I always used to hope the switchboard would put me through to you.'

Our eyes meet, and the memory of his whipped-cream phone voice flows back to me. I feel an irrational twinge of guilt now, for always having passed him on to one of my salivating single colleagues.

I knock back my first shot. 'Okay. Return confession. The women in my department used to fight over who got to speak with you, whenever you called.'

Oliver appears, understandably, fairly delighted by this. He leans back against the booth we're in, stretching out his long legs. He is wearing a designer shirt, but somehow it looks much less ostentatious on him than I suspect it would on Lawrence. 'And were you . . . one of them?'

I shake my head apologetically. 'Sorry. I was married.'

Actually, that's not quite accurate, I should add. *I'm still married.*

'Tell me about him. Emma's father.'

I open my mouth to correct him, then change my mind. I'm not sure why, exactly. 'We rushed things. Don't get me wrong – I wouldn't change having Emma for the world. But Lawrence and I . . . we were never a great match.'

'It happens,' he says sympathetically. 'But hey – you got your beautiful little girl, right?'

I agree with a smile. 'I take it you never had any of your own? Kids, I mean.'

'Ah, no. I always wanted to – just never met the right person, I guess.' He smiles too, but a little wistfully. 'Or maybe I did, but not at the right time. It's a funny thing, getting older, isn't it?'

I push a sudden pulse of Josh from my mind. 'You can't be much older than me.'

'Forty-two? And obviously, I know that's not *old*. But still. The idea that I might never have kids of my own ...' He shakes his head. 'It's just a bit weird.'

'I get that. I thought the same once, too.'

He looks pensive. 'So, what you're saying is, don't give up?'

'Sorry,' I say, feeling chastened. 'Didn't mean to patronise.'

'No, gosh, you didn't. I genuinely can't hear that enough.'

I wonder, suddenly, if this is his deal-breaker: that he wants to have kids. If that is his red line, dating-wise. I can't probe him on it, though. We have done nothing more than share some erotically themed drinks. It would feel way too presumptuous to ask if I should walk away now, because one day he will want to start a family – and I cannot promise him that I will, too. It's simply not something I've had to think about, ever since having Emma and splitting up with Lawrence.

But there is something I need to make clear – even at the risk of firmly killing the mood. *I should put my cards on the table, Oliver. I'm not really looking for anything at the moment. I'm just so busy, with work and my daughter ...*

Because that, actually, is the truth. I just can't picture how I would find the time to fit a relationship into my life as it stands.

Something else is also true, though. Which is that I do not, in fact, want to say any of that right now. Because I have really missed dressing up and drinking silly cocktails and flirting with a handsome man and feeling desired.

Later, in the cold at the cab rank, Oliver kisses me, his lips laced with Kahlúa and raspberry from the cocktails. He slips a hand through my hair, ribboning it between his fingers, his body inching in as the kiss starts to deepen.

I have missed my moment, I realise, to warn him I am everything he is not looking for. I should have been upfront about that from the start. But I wonder, now, if it even matters. If we might not have ended up doing this anyway.

Three taxis come and go, and I'm chilled to the bone by the time I eventually make it home. But for the rest of the weekend I cannot stop smiling, and checking my phone.

50.

Josh

December 2007

'Wilf? *Wilf*. For Christ's sake, I know you're in there.'

After five minutes of banging on Wilf's front door and disturbing his neighbours and attempting to say, *It's okay, I'm a friend* in Spanish, it inches open, just a crack.

'Go away.'

'I can't,' I say, resisting the urge to shoulder-barge my way in. 'I'd have to catch a plane. And I'm not doing that for another forty-eight hours.'

'I don't want to see you. I've put all that stuff behind me, Josh.' Wilf lowers his voice to a hiss. 'Do you know how hard it was for me to hide from them?'

'Yes, because it's taken me this long to track you down.'

In the end – and I will never admit this to a soul, not even Rachel – I paid a private investigator an extortionate amount of money to do in a matter of weeks what I'd failed to do in four years.

I doubted the guy at first. Told him all about Wilf's IQ, then grilled him on exactly how he planned to find him. To which he said in a withering monotone, 'Does he cope well with uncertainty? Can he deal with a life entirely lacking in routine?'

'Er, no. The opposite, actually.'

'Then that Mensa membership means fuck all, mate.'

* * *

As soon as Wilf lets me in, my relief pivots without warning to anger. So much time spent worrying about his welfare, being stalked in my own home, abruptly cut off and unable to talk to him. I shove him, hard, both hands to his chest. 'You fucking abandoned me.'

Red-faced, and apparently equally furious, Wilf shoves me back, with surprising force. I have to grab the edge of the doorway to keep my footing.

I straighten up and we regard each other, breathing hard. It's my move, now, apparently.

Tension sharpens the space between us. For a moment, this could go either way.

No. I shudder out a breath, turn my back. I didn't come all the way out here to have a fist fight with the guy who saved my life.

Without invitation I move into Wilf's living room, the ceramic tiles chilling my feet through my socks. 'Seriously, did our friendship mean nothing to you? You knew people were after me and you slunk away like a fucking coward. They broke into my flat three times. I was followed home from work, I got silent phone calls—'

'That's why I *left*, you idiot.'

I turn to face him. 'What?'

'They gave up after that, no?'

I sit down on his sofa, put my head in my hands. The rage has begun to recede. 'I've been *worried* about you. I thought you were dead.'

'No, you didn't.' He straightens the collar of his polo shirt. 'You knew I'd gone into hiding. Why the hell else would you pay a private investigator to track me down?'

I sigh guiltily. 'How did you know?'

'Because he was an amateur.' Wilf rolls his eyes. 'I'd save your money in future.'

'He found you in about five minutes.'

'Not very subtly. Was he a trainee?'

'Why are you being an arsehole?'

Flush-cheeked, he spreads his hands. '*Because*. I had a good life, Josh. None of this had to happen. I was only trying to do you a favour.'

'It's not my fault if you failed to cover your tracks at work.'

'I didn't fail,' he snaps. 'I was considering pitching it, remember?'

My heart is still pumping hard, from relief, or anger, who knows. 'Okay, then it's not my fault you changed your mind.'

He flops heavily down on the sofa next to me, then – to my bemusement – pulls a pack of cigarettes and lighter from his pocket.

'What the hell are you doing?'

He shrugs. 'Tar's transient now. They can't kill me.'

I take him in for a couple of moments. And, perhaps for the first time, it occurs to me that his youthfulness does hint at a kind of invincibility. It's over four years since I've seen him, and nearly eight since we took that pill. And he hasn't aged a day. The thought is unsurprising and staggering, all at once.

I never doubted Wilf's genius. Not in my gut. But, even now, I don't think I've fully processed the enormity of what he invented. Of what we did.

Still. Guilt-free smoking seems dubious, as perks go.

'Transient tar,' I say. 'Yeah, I can definitely see the appeal.'

Wilf lights up, exhales a plume of smoke, then offers the packet to me.

'No, I was . . . Never mind.' I shake my head. 'Am I allowed to ask how you're surviving, these days?'

'I play poker.'

I almost laugh, but save it just in time. 'Really? For money?'

He nods. 'Turns out I'm quite good.'

I enjoy for a moment the idea of someone sitting down with Wilf for a game of poker, believing they have even the remotest chance of outmanoeuvring Mr Mensa.

'Can you even speak Spanish?'

He looks at me witheringly. 'Yes, fluently. I learnt when I was ten.'

Of course you did.

Through his open window I can see a raft of rooftops, the silver score of Mediterranean on the horizon. The weather's in the low twenties, the air blue and breezeless. A world away from the slate skies and unbroken gloom of home.

'Wilf,' I say, after a while. 'I wanted to ask . . . if there's any chance the pill can be reversed.'

He takes a few moments to respond. 'Is that why you're really here?'

Up to a point, perhaps. But it wasn't my sole motivation. 'No. I wanted to see *you*. To check you were okay. Like I've been trying to do for the past four years.'

'Fine.' He drags then exhales, shakes his head. 'You can't reverse the effects. I did make it clear they'd be permanent.'

I try to ignore the wrenching feeling inside me, as if someone is trying to crowbar my heart from my body. 'But that was nearly eight years ago. Could the science not have moved on since then?'

'You're forgetting that "the science" doesn't technically exist, Josh.'

'It does in your brain. Please, Wilf.'

'What – you want me to mix something up in my rented kitchen-cum-pharmaceutical lab?'

'Just tell me if it can be done.'

He retrieves an ashtray from the floor, taps a long worm of ash into it. 'Is this to do with Rachel?'

'Partly,' I admit.

After Rachel made it clear – again – that she wasn't interested in taking the second pill, my mind drifted once more to the idea of reversal.

I think this might be my only chance, Wilf.

'Are you saying you regret taking it?' He sounds indignant, as though I flew all the way out here with the sole aim of affronting his genius.

I frown. 'It's not as simple as that. I'm grateful it saved me, but . . .' It's hard to admit I've been questioning again lately the reality of that long-ago fear. Whether it was all in my head. A bit like waking in the night to see a hooded figure in your bedroom, then snapping on the light to realise it's just a chair piled with clothes. 'Sometimes I think that if I'd just hung on, everything would have been okay.'

Wilf shrugs. 'Or you might be dead in a box.'

Touché.

'Do you ever worry about the future?' I ask him.

'What about it?'

It's hard to articulate, exactly. The idea of still being here a hundred years from now, all the people I love, dead. Just me and Wilf . . . doing what, exactly? What if we are both tired of living by then?

It's ironic, I sometimes think. That I swapped fearing one future for another.

So maybe the hard truth of life is that there is always something to fear.

It's not long before Wilf asks me to leave. He says he's got things to do, poker to play. I decide to comply, since my vision of sitting reconciled together in pavement cafés was evidently just fantasy.

I can't stay here any longer. I feel too bruised to hang around. So I buy an extortionately priced last-minute plane ticket home, then head to a beach bar to fill my last few hours of time. I take an outside table, order a *vino tinto* and watch the sun melt into the Mediterranean. The fronds of the palm trees turn to flames, the warm air cooling against my arms.

Of course, I then get drunk, miss my flight and kiss goodbye to hundreds of euros I did not have. I end up aimlessly wandering the back streets of Torrevieja as the alcohol burns off and its various toxic by-products kick in.

At the airport the next morning, while I'm waiting to board the third flight to Luton I've now bought a ticket for, a message comes up on my phone from an unknown number.

> Try Hester Carver, if you must. She's the only person I trust. But you'd need to give her the other pill.
> Assuming Rachel hasn't taken it.

Head pounding, I text a reply – saying thank you and sorry – but my message bounces straight back.

51.

Rachel

August 2003

There was one time, when I was dating Lawrence, that I thought about asking Josh if we could try again.

It was August, two nights after Lawrence had overheard me telling Josh we were only a casual thing.

I rang Josh's doorbell in the middle of a thunderstorm.

He didn't say anything when he opened the door, just stepped aside to let me in. I was soaked through, without a coat or umbrella, my clothes moulded like fresh plaster to my skin. The rain had been a shock, but in a good way. A heavy, cathartic blast. I hoped clarity would follow.

'Lawrence left,' I said, after a couple of moments.

He nodded. 'I mean, you hung up then switched your phone off. So I guessed it probably wasn't good.'

'Josh, I think . . .'

'You think what?' he said, fixing me with his dark, patient eyes.

But I found I couldn't say what I'd gone there to say. *I think I made a mistake.* Because I knew that before I said those words, I had to be sure.

And I wasn't, not completely.

A few things had changed at the flat, in the two years since I'd left. Décor and some furniture, our wedding photo no longer in the living room. But, small alterations aside, I knew the beating heart of the home we'd once shared was exactly the same. The slant of the light, the laboured clunk of the pipes. I pressed a foot to the floorboards, to feel their familiar creak. The air smelt the same, too, of hand soap and soft pillows and Josh.

As he fetched towels and clean clothes for me to change into, I told him more about the fight I'd had with Lawrence.

'Sorry,' he said, reaching for a bottle of brandy, after I'd dried off and got dressed. 'Kind of feels like it's my fault.'

I shook my head. 'No, it's . . . I think we crossed wires. Me and Lawrence.'

'In what way?'

'He says he loves me.'

Josh didn't reply for a while. He just measured out two fingers, passed me a glass. Then: 'And you don't love him?'

I hesitated, then said, 'Sorry. I shouldn't be talking to you about this.'

He didn't comment, just poured one for himself, knocked it back.

I took him in for a moment – his jeans and creased T-shirt, his bare feet, the dark tidemark of his never-changing stubble. So different from Lawrence, who was always pristine in a way that came naturally to him but not me. He ironed everything – socks, boxers, bed sheets – and wore shoes indoors. Sometimes, he didn't take off his work clothes until we went to bed.

Right then, Josh's crumpled imperfection made me ache. I wanted to sink into it, shut my eyes and stay there.

'Sometimes, when Lawrence is saying he loves me, it's almost like . . . he's actually trying to control me. Does that make sense?'

Josh nodded, but said, 'At the end of the day, I don't know him, Rach.'

I apologised again, though it came out as more of a gasp. As if I couldn't believe I could be this confused.

'Rachel. Don't take this the wrong way. But why are you here?'

The question was gentle yet exposing. Like a breath parting water.

I suspected he was wondering why I wasn't with Ingrid, or Polly, or Lola, or anyone else who didn't have good reason to occasionally fantasise about Lawrence's funeral.

'I wanted a friend.' Somehow, this felt like both the fairest and most cruel thing I could have said to him in that moment.

Outside, rain was twisting from the sky, battering the windows, relentless.

There didn't seem to be an immediate solution to the Lawrence predicament, so we just kept drinking. Eventually, between us, we sank the bottle, and that was the point at which my memories blacked out.

The next morning, I woke with a stiff neck, alone in Josh's bed.

Panic rose. I lifted the duvet.

Fully clothed.

Thank God.

Yes, Lawrence and I were having problems – but it wouldn't have excused me doing that.

I lay there for a few moments, breathing in the scent of Josh from where it lingered on his bedding. Through the unlatched window the outside air felt clear, washed clean by last night's rain.

On the wall facing Josh's bed, there were a few patches of emulsion in varying shades of vanilla, painted over the pale blue. He must have been thinking about redecorating.

I sat up and pushed back my hair. On Josh's nightstand, I noticed a copy of *The Remains of the Day*, the page turned down about halfway through.

I heard footsteps approaching. Then Josh appeared in the doorway, slim and quiet, like a shadow.

'It's okay,' he said, before I could say anything. 'I slept on the sofa. In all my clothes.' He smiled. 'Even socks.'

It used to be our running joke that we could never have sex with socks on. Even if the moment had taken us and we were still partly clothed, it had always been our agreed red line: all socks *had* to come off.

'That's good,' I said meekly, feeling like the world's worst human. My mouth tasted of stagnant brandy.

'Yeah, that wouldn't have been such a great idea, would it?'

I shook my head, and a mud weight of silence sank through the room. Feeling the immediate need to counter it, I nodded at the paint samples on the wall. 'Top left looks best.'

He laughed, loosely. 'Can't even remember which was which now. I kind of . . . ran out of steam.'

Our eyes met, and sadness cut through me, sharp and deep as the slice of a knife.

I took a breath. 'I'm sorry I came here last night. Complaining about Lawrence. That was spectacularly unfair.'

He rubbed his jaw. 'Maybe. A bit.'

'If it helps, I feel terrible.'

'Body or soul?'

'God, both.'

'I'll make some coffee.'

Another pause, and there was something inside me that wanted to prolong the moment, for the seconds to slow.

I nodded down at *The Remains of the Day* on his nightstand. 'Any good?'

A beat. 'Yeah. It's . . . all right.'

'What's it about?' I lifted it up, flipping it briefly over. 'The war?'

Something softened in his eyes, and he shot me a smile. 'Um, kind of. Yeah.'

As he turned to leave the room, he paused by the door. 'Rach, for what it's worth, I don't think you should be with someone who tries to control you.'

My whole body agreed, when he said that. But it would take another year before I acted on what I already knew.

52.

Josh

December 2007

Just before Christmas, I meet Oliver for the first time.

I've been expecting for a while to encounter the new boyfriend Rachel's been seeing since late summer. But up till now she has somehow succeeded in keeping the two of us apart.

They're the final ones of our group to show up to the pub, taking seats at the other end of our run of tables. But as soon as it's my round, they follow me to the bar.

Oliver is tall, and – to my surprise – silver-haired. He's very smartly turned out, and I get the feeling he's exacting. The kind of guy who disinfects his groceries, sets a timer to brush his teeth, routinely tests his fog light.

He has his arm around her waist. She looks ethereally beautiful, in a kelp-green sweater, blonde hair cascading over the front of her shoulder. I can't deny that he and Rachel look good together. You'd see them and think, *What a nice couple*.

I sometimes try to work out if Rachel looks noticeably older than me now. If, standing side by side, we appear in any way odd. But it's a question I will always struggle to answer. Because, to my mind, she is just Rachel.

As she introduces us, it occurs to me that Oliver could be Lawrence's slightly squarer older brother. I guess she's developed a type since we split up, though I'm not too sure what this says about me.

'Oliver Danvers,' he says, pumping my hand so hard, I can't work out if he's trying to alpha-male me or is genuinely enthused to meet me.

The urge to reply with *Joshua Foster* is fierce. I'm pretty sure the me of a few years ago wouldn't have hesitated. But I decide Rachel would probably appreciate it if I didn't make this into a rutting stags thing. 'Josh. Hi. Good to meet you.'

Then, for reasons best known to herself, Rachel says she'll get the next round in and moves a little further along the bar, leaving her husband and her new boyfriend to arm-wrestle their way out of the world's most awkward silence.

'Rachel tells me you're a teacher.'

Straight for the jugular, then.

'I write novels as well. Kind of juggle the two.'

A lofty smile. 'When were you last published?'

I scratch an itch that isn't there on my jawline. 'Four years ago. Or thereabouts. They take a while to . . . gestate.'

He nods, thoughtfully. 'A bloke I used to work with is a writer now. He's on a crazy schedule. Bangs one out every year.'

The pub is loud and busy and hot. I feel as if the whole world is ringing in my ears.

'Great. Does he? Great.'

'Do you write under a pseudonym?'

It's not hard to work out where this is going. 'Nope. My own name.'

'Oh.' He affects surprise. 'I don't think I've ever heard of you.'

I lift my left hand then to rub my chin, so he gets a good view of my wedding ring. This is petty, I know. But – for a moment, at least – it makes me feel marginally better.

Averting his gaze from my hand, Oliver lowers his voice and says, with a wink, 'Listen, I own a recruitment business. So if you're ever in need of work, let me know. We have all sorts of openings that could suit you.'

He stops just short of saying, *slaughterhouse operative*, or *cold-caller of the elderly*, which would have fully outed him as the arsehole I know him to be.

At this point, Rachel returns, handing over our drinks, and she looks so bright and hopeful and happy, it breaks my heart a little bit.

Back at the flat, in a kind of remote toast to Wilf, I decide to smoke a cigarette. It's been years since I've done so, social smoking at college like everybody does. But I bought a pack from the corner shop on my way home, because, tonight, I fancied it.

Tar's transient now. Fuck it, they can't kill me. May as well enjoy having vices.

I light up in bed, then send Rachel a text.

> Have to say, I'm not a fan

> Okay

> Don't want to sound bitter, but you can do better

> You don't know him

> Do you??

> I'm sorry if he made you feel uncomfortable

> He didn't. But it should worry you that he tried.

She doesn't reply.

53.

Rachel

December 2007

One evening close to Christmas, Oliver and I have just got home from a night out with Giles and Lola when he says, 'Can I ask you something? It's about Josh.'

I make us both a mint tea while Oliver switches on a lamp, flips through my CDs. There is no jazz, so he picks blues, an album that probably once belonged to Lawrence.

Oliver and Josh met for the first time in the pub a couple of nights ago. Just briefly, while we were all at the bar. An encounter so fleeting that neither of us even mentioned it afterwards.

But Josh texted that night, to let me know exactly what he thought of Oliver. I read his messages, surprised to see they were uncharacteristically acerbic, then deleted them straight away.

'Giles mentioned something earlier, about Josh being twenty-nine,' Oliver says from the sofa, as I pass him his tea. 'I said I thought he was your age, then he got all flustered and told me to talk to you about it.'

I sit down next to him. It's actually surprising, to be honest, that all this hasn't come out before tonight, given that we've been seeing each other for nearly three months now.

'You're thirty-seven,' Oliver prompts, as if he thinks I might have forgotten.

'I know,' I say, with a loose smile.

'Okay, I mean, hardly an enormous age gap,' he says slowly. 'But there's obviously something going on here. Can you fill me in?'

So I do, because it's only fair. I tell him everything, apart from where Josh got the pill.

Oliver listens intently the whole time I'm talking, never taking his eyes off me. When I'm done, he leans back on the sofa and clips out a breath, loosens his shirt collar. 'So Josh is actually your age, chronologically. But he looks twenty-nine, and will do for the rest of his life?'

'Yep.'

'Wow. Talk about a head-fuck.' He glances over at me. 'That's why you left?'

I nod.

'You should have stayed. Had yourself a toy-boy.'

I swallow. 'That's not funny.'

There's a slight chill to the air now. I reach to the back of the sofa, pull Emma's Peppa Pig blanket over my knees.

'Sorry,' he says. 'Look, for what it's worth, I actually agree with your stance. You'd be mad to take a pill like that. I can't think of anything more horrifying than living indefinitely, frankly.'

I don't comment on this. 'I'm sorry I didn't tell you before.'

'Why didn't you, out of interest?'

I'm not even sure myself.

I had told him Josh was my first love. But not what it meant.

I shrug softly. 'It's a difficult thing to know how to explain. And it caused a few issues, with Lawrence. I didn't want it to cause any with us.'

He appears to consider this. 'Honesty's a real thing for me, Rachel. With my last girlfriend—'

'I know, and I'm sorry.' Heart contracting with guilt, I reach for his hand, take it tightly in mine. 'It just felt easier not to tell you at first, and then—'

'Or maybe you thought we would never come to anything.'

I recoil a little, my hand loosening.

'Sorry. Sorry. That was ...' Briefly, he shuts his eyes. 'I guess this is all just a bit ... I mean, the man's hardly a one out of ten, is he?'

This surprises me. Oliver's always struck me as fairly robust on that front, not prone to self-doubt, or lacking confidence in his appearance.

'Looks aren't everything,' I say, then feel instantly bad, prepare to gabble a backtrack.

He doesn't appear to have taken offence, though. 'True. And you know what they say. Your first love is never your true love.'

I've never heard that before. But I don't tell him so.

'So, do you really think the pill has worked?'

I stare into my tea, permitting myself to briefly picture Josh, that stopped clock gifting him with the same taut skin and bright eyes, lean build and dark hair as he had nearly a decade ago. 'Yes, I think so.'

'Can I ask you something?'

'Of course.'

'If Josh found a way to reverse the effects of it, what would you do?'

Oliver's storm-grey eyes are fixed on me, unblinking. It's clear I cannot risk hesitating, a pause of any kind.

'Nothing. I wouldn't do anything. It's *you* I want, Oliver.'

'You're sure about that?'

'I'm sure,' I murmur before leaning forward, putting my lips to his. 'I'm sure, and I'm sorry.'

Oliver is, I have discovered, an old-school romantic. He likes to kiss in cinemas and parks, linger in art galleries with our arms snaked around each other. We go to see live blues and jazz bands, eat fish and chips by the river. Often I fall asleep by his side, my head on his shoulder. He drops food to my doorstep, if it's late and I have Emma, and I thank him with a kiss, my back against the brickwork, that singular pleasure of wanting him, yet knowing I have to wait.

I spend much of my time like this, longing for more of him. Once or twice he has called late at night, to tell me he's been thinking about me. And we talk a little, the conversation slowly growing heated and intimate. Then, after we hang up and I am alone in bed, I find myself unable to stop thinking of him, too.

It's funny, really. That the running joke in my office about Oliver's phone voice has become – quite out of nowhere – my reality.

Not long after Christmas, I introduce him to Emma. He has asked to meet her before, but up till now I've said no. I'm pretty sure my only hesitation comes from knowing what is at stake here. Emma is deep-feeling and sensitive, and, if she and Oliver don't hit it off, I'm not sure how he and I could ever continue. It's felt less risky, so far, to keep them apart.

In the end, though, the occasion of their meeting turns out to be beautifully unexceptional. We arrange for him to come over one night between Christmas and the new year. And he handles the whole thing perfectly. From the moment he walks through the door, Emma accepts him as a friend.

We watch *Beauty and the Beast*, the three of us cosy on the sofa, sharing a bowl of popcorn. Oliver asks Emma lots of affable questions about pre-school and her favourite teachers, books she likes to read, her swimming classes and what she got for Christmas. She tells him about my dad, and the balance bike he gave her, and what we ate for breakfast on Christmas Day – piles of pancakes, towering with toppings, which she's been talking about in roughly five-minute increments ever since.

The next morning, Emma and I find Oliver in the kitchen, flipping pancakes. He asks her what toppings she would like, and she suggests marshmallows, Nutella and banana. Oliver agrees this is an excellent combination.

I stand and watch them for a few moments, my new boyfriend and my daughter, having a conversation I know she will never remember. But one that I will, for the rest of my life.

For the first time in a long while, I feel my heart relax.

It's all going to work out.

Just stay away from Josh, I think, *and everything will be okay.*

54.

Josh

March 2008

'Good news?' enquires a soft voice behind me.

I snap my laptop closed.

'What's that about a pill?'

'Nothing,' I bristle. 'It's private.'

Sitting up in her bed, Charley scratches her long neck, the same neck I was kissing less than five minutes ago. She says nothing.

Briefly, I shut my eyes. 'Sorry. Sorry.'

She shrugs as I look over at her. Light is lancing through her bedroom blinds. She is slight and startlingly pretty, with a dark pixie cut and huge, expressive eyes.

For a moment, I imagine — as I sometimes do when I meet someone new — telling the truth. Confessing that, in fact, I am nearly a whole decade older than she thinks I am, and then explaining why.

But I resist the urge to get into that conversation, which would be long and complicated, and would also — I'm fairly sure — paint me as the guy who took a pill so he could trick women into bed.

Last night went pretty much how these encounters always do, for me. Surface-level pleasure. No real connection, or sense of a spark that might endure. She told me about her job at the Serious Fraud Office — ironically enough — and I ran her through what I enjoyed about being a writer, a reader, a half-decent cook. I sprinkled a few jokes in there too, so as not to bore her stupid, though the jury's probably still out on that.

Charley leans over to take the cigarette I've half-smoked from between my fingers. 'I think you should probably go now, Josh. I've got work to do.'

This is the first time I've seen Charley, but I already know it will also be the last.

Is this how it's always going to be now? Unable to get close to anyone, because of the secret I am keeping?

Most likely, unless I start telling the truth, which I've no plans to do. So I simply nod and pull on my T-shirt, find my jacket. Cast around for my wallet and phone. Check my watch is still on my wrist.

Just before I leave, I hesitate.

'Absolutely *not*,' Charley says, pre-empting any parting acts of idiocy from me, like suggesting we hug goodbye.

Outside, while I'm waiting for my cab, I dial the number for Wilf's old colleague Hester. She gave it to me in her email responding to the tentative enquiry about an antidote it took me a full three months to work up to making.

I googled her first. She was young and pretty, a Cambridge-educated scientist, like Wilf. It occurred to me that perhaps she was his crustacean-averse date from Valentine's night, that time.

But as soon as Hester says, 'Hello?' I hang up.

There is something inside me that just needs to check with Rachel, one final time, that she doesn't want the pill. After that, I can hand it over to Hester – who would need it, apparently, in order to develop anything new – and let it disappear for good.

* * *

I text Rachel, ask to meet for a coffee. She doesn't reply for a while, and then there's a bit of back and forth, as she's generally pretty stacked, between work and Oliver and Emma and dealing with Lawrence's ever-more mercurial moods. But eventually we settle on a time.

She turns up late, breathless with apologies.

The first thing I say is, 'I should be the one apologising. For sending you those texts, about Oliver.'

I regretted them almost instantly. It wasn't my place, I realised, to vet him for her. If he'd threatened me with a hammer, that might have been different. But in reality he had only raised his hackles slightly. And who knows – I might have behaved similarly, in his position.

Rachel smiles as if she's still slightly baffled by them. 'I'd love to know what he said to you.'

'Forget it. I was being oversensitive.' I mean, I could tell her, but to what end?

Instead, I ask her how work's going. She's been a professional artist for a few years now, and is already so busy she has a waiting list for commissions. I no longer see that drained expression she so often wore on a Friday night, though it always seemed more like ennui than actual exhaustion. Her cheeks are a little fuller these days. Yet somehow, to me, she appears lighter.

She tells me she's renting a studio space in town, that it's no longer practical for her to work from home, with a toddler running around and white spirit and wet canvases everywhere. 'I've lost count of the number of elbow patches I've given my clothes.'

'Bet you never look back,' I say.

She laughs in agreement. 'How many minutes of my life do you think I wasted in meetings talking about people analytics and employment law?'

'Doesn't matter. You're doing it now. That's what counts.'

'Not if you ask Lawrence.'

I've trained myself not to comment on all the crappy things Lawrence keeps insisting on saying to Rachel. One: I'm not a parent, so I do get that there are dynamics involved between them that I will never understand. Two: it only makes me look – and feel – bitter. And I'm not so arrogant as to assume that a few offhand comments from me will be in any way useful to Rachel. The best thing I can do, I have learned, is just listen, and be there for her.

I summon the good grace to ask after Oliver, at which she moves her gaze to the window, towards the sunless sky. To her credit, I think she tries hard to de-giddy her smile. But some sentiments you can't suppress. 'He's good. We're good.'

'I'm pleased for you.' And, though she probably doesn't believe me, it isn't a lie. Because I've only ever wanted her to be happy.

We chat for a few minutes more, then I say, 'Rach, I've got something to tell you. I've been in touch with an old colleague of Wilf's about a possible antidote. She's willing to meet me. But she would need the second pill, and—'

'What?' Rachel's brown eyes become suddenly brittle. 'Why are you telling me this?'

'Because I wanted to check—'

'I don't want to talk about that pill with you any more.' She swigs back the last of her coffee, the skin on her neck flushing pink, and zips her bag with a brusqueness I can tell she wants me to feel. 'Even if you do find an antidote, or some way to reverse it, I'm telling you: I don't want to know.'

As her voice recedes, the burning feeling in me stays. The sting of her words, left lodged beneath my skin.

'I can't live in limbo any more,' she whispers. 'It's not fair. I don't want to be ninety and still thinking about you, Josh.'

She's right, I realise, remorse rolling through me. Of course she is. How can I possibly say I'm happy for her, then keep trying to pull her back to the past, whatever my motivations?

'I'm sorry,' I manage, eventually.

'I feel bad saying that. But I've moved on now. And you should probably do the same.'

55.

Rachel

December 2010

A few days before Christmas, Emma and I head to London for some last-minute shopping. After several frantic months working on commissions, I've finally signed off for the festive season. This is something I am steadfast on: a fortnight of quality time at Christmas, every single year, for me and my daughter.

Josh is in London today too, seeing his agent and publisher. We agree to meet rinkside at Somerset House for hot chocolates, to watch the skating.

I haven't spent time with him one-on-one for eighteen months or so, since that day at the café, when he told me he was still hoping to find an antidote to the pill. But I agreed to meet him today – with Oliver's full knowledge – because there is something I need to ask him.

But, so far, I've found it too hard to say the words.

It is close to five o'clock. The courtyard glints gold in the dusk, shimmering with Christmas and whirling with skaters. Next to me, my six-year-old is watching it all, mesmerised. Her blonde hair is wild and haphazard, in desperate need of a trim, and her mouth is smeared with hot chocolate, which has also found its way on to the front of her pale grey coat. Lawrence occasionally gets huffy about what he sees as her scruffiness. But I am determined never to get hung up on hairbrushes and wet wipes and on only letting her eat stuff that won't stain. Because it is moments like these – messy or not – that I cherish the most, that I use to plug the ache in me whenever we are apart.

Josh turns to look at me, the rosy glow of the rink reflected in his eyes, breath clouding in the rimy air. His skin is so flawless, it gleams. He told me once he can't shave any more, because it won't grow back. But I'm secretly pleased by this, because I've always thought stubble looks lovely on him.

I have known for a while that it can no longer be in question: a decade on, and he hasn't aged a day. He will look, for the rest of his life, as though the best is yet to come.

In contrast, I'm aware that tiny lines spring to my eyes and mouth now, whenever I smile. That my skin has a touch less spring these days, and my clothes are a little snugger. I'm not sure if this bothers me, really. I certainly don't expend much energy thinking about it. But, whenever I am with Josh, it's hard not to compare the way I look with the appearance of a man who is, essentially, living life in freeze-frame.

He tells me about the meeting he's had today, to discuss a potential project. His publisher has come up with an idea for a novel, and asked Josh if he will write it. 'I know beggars can't be choosers, but the idea was pretty bonkers.'

At this, Emma giggles.

'What's funny?' Josh says, turning to her with a teasing expression. 'Bonkers? What's so funny about bonkers?'

This, of course, only makes her laugh harder.

'So will you do it?' I ask.

He nods, but so sadly it hurts my heart. 'Can't not write. Or turn down work. If that's my only option then ... of course.'

'Have faith,' I assure him. 'I'm sure world domination is just around the corner.'

He smiles gratefully. 'So, tell me. How's everything going, with Oliver?'

I struggle to know how to answer this. Because there will never be an easy way to talk about my boyfriend with the man I once promised to love forever.

I let out a breath, nodding down at Emma. She has returned her attention to her hot chocolate, clamping the cup over her nose, determined to fish out every last drop with her tongue. 'Can I fill you in later?'

'Sure. Sorry.' He nods back, then claps his hands. 'Right. Who's up for a skate?'

Emma immediately abandons her cup. 'Me!'

'No one?' Josh says, pretending to look around. 'You're sure? No one else wants to come skating with me?'

'Me!' Emma squeals. 'I do!'

Josh exaggerates a shrug. 'Oh, well. I guess it's just me, then.'

Emma tugs fiercely at his coat between gulps of laughter, practically falling off her seat in desperation. 'Me, I want to!'

He looks down at her. 'Oh, hello. Didn't see you there.'

This elicits another feverish round of giggles, which makes me laugh too.

Josh dips his face to Emma's. 'Did I hear you say you'd like to come skating with me?'

She nods several times in quick succession.

He looks at me. 'Coming?'

The truth is, I would love to get on the rink right now. But I am a terrible skater, all legs and no co-ordination, even more so than Josh. Which means that at some point I will be forced to grab his hand. And that – at Christmas, on an ice rink together – would be crossing the line I have drawn inside my heart.

I shake my head, lift my sketchbook. 'I'm recording it all for posterity.'

Josh looks down at Emma. 'It's just you and me, kid. Mum's bottled it.'

'Here, sweetie.' I take out a tissue and wipe the chocolate from Emma's mouth and chin before they go. Over the top of her head, I meet Josh's eye, and feel his gaze tug at me, like a tide running out to sea.

'Come on, then,' he says to Emma, taking her mittened hand. 'Better get . . .' He pauses, raising his eyebrows at her in anticipation.

'. . . our skates on!' she squeals, delightedly.

I have worried since Emma was born that it is cruel, asking Josh if he would like to spend time with her. That I am parading parenthood in front of him. It often feels, at the very least, spectacularly insensitive.

But, whenever we are all together, those misgivings just melt away.

As they walk off hand in hand towards the ice rink, Josh bending down to hear something Emma is saying, I have to swallow a lump in my throat so large, it almost won't shift.

56.

Rachel

December 2010

Back at home, after Emma goes to bed, I crack open the box of mince pies I picked up in Fortnum & Mason, because Ingrid goes on about them every year as if they've been handcrafted by Jesus Christ himself. And then I decide to watch *The Holiday*, because there is no better Christmas film. Last night I suggested to Oliver that we put it on, at which he pulled a face and said, 'You must have seen it a hundred times. And I have to say, I never did quite get the hype.'

But he is out tonight, at a Christmas cheese-and-wine do with clients.

We moved in together last year, into a gated estate he'd had his eye on for a while. Emma loves it, and has already made friends with all the neighbours' kids, because she is just that kind of girl. Open-hearted and curious, fun-seeking. Oliver bought her a new bike as a moving-in present, and she has been wobbling up and down the road on it most evenings, pink-cheeked with pride, even if she's tumbled and scraped a knee.

The rent is eye-watering, though, and the house does lack a little character. I think that is what I will always miss most about the flat I shared with Josh. The quirks I ended up growing to love. The tilt of the light through our wonky front window, the constantly clunking pipes, the creak of oak beneath my feet.

But life now is about my humans, not a house – coming downstairs after a long day in my home studio to find Oliver at the kitchen table, patiently talking Emma through the basics of fractions. Having the space, at last, to host barbecues and dinner parties and just-because get-togethers. Hearing the murmur of Oliver's voice through the kitchen ceiling at bedtime, as he and Emma read *The Wind in the Willows*, or *Charlotte's Web*. And our new tradition of messy, rambling Sunday-night suppers after Lawrence has dropped Emma home. The family life that for so long lived only in my imagination.

From the outset, Oliver never seemed to irritate Lawrence in quite the same way that Josh did. They bonded fairly quickly over work, and sometimes Oliver cracks a niche joke about tax deductibles or the stock market that Lawrence seems to appreciate. They'll never be best buddies, obviously. But I feel pretty lucky that, for now, relations between them appear to be harmonious.

And I've been enjoying having Oliver to myself more now, too. The pleasure of eating breakfast in bed together on Saturdays, strong coffee and fried eggs on toast. The everyday novelty of curling up in his arms and watching *Sherlock*, or *Spooks*. Deciding it would definitely be good karma, to christen every room in our first family home. Last night, we found ourselves having sex in the downstairs cloakroom because we were in an empty house with a free fifteen minutes, the ensuing fuck so intense my legs began to shake.

As *The Holiday* finishes, it starts to snow outside, the usually bright light from the street lamp turned blurry by a torrent of white.

There isn't a real fireplace here, but the gas one is quite pretty. I switch it on and watch the flames dance, as if to music. And then I call him.

'Josh.' I'm just going to come out with it now. The words have been sitting like stones in my stomach all day. 'I couldn't say this in front of Emma. But ... I think we should get divorced.'

There follows a subdued pause, during which I hear what I think is – bizarrely – the click of a cigarette lighter.

'Are you *smoking*?'

'Only now and then. The tar can't kill me.'

I consider this. 'Seems like flimsy reasoning.'

'They do relax me, annoyingly enough.' I hear him take a drag. 'So, are you going to marry Oliver?'

I shift my gaze to the bright confetti of the snowstorm beyond the window. 'I don't think so. But I do think it probably makes him uncomfortable.'

'That we were once together?'

'That we're still married. Do you blame him?'

'For what specifically?'

'For feeling awkward. About us.'

I don't tell him – because of course I cannot – that a couple of months ago Oliver and I agreed to start trying for a baby. I'd expected the right decision about having more children to alight, at some point, in my heart. I thought I'd wake up one day and just *know*. But, in the end, it felt more rational than that. What it came down to, I concluded, was that they would both be brilliant: Emma as a big sister, and Oliver as a dad. Our family would be like a rose bush in a garden, becoming only more beautiful with each new bloom.

Having a baby with Lawrence was a leap of faith, in many ways. But the idea of doing it with Oliver feels exactly the opposite. A soft landing, well mapped-out, the safest of bets.

Josh knocks out what I imagine to be a smoky breath. 'Okay. Well, I have no idea how to get divorced, but I'm sure Oliver will have the relevant paperwork ready and waiting.'

'Please don't give me a hard time about this. I'm not sure I have the mental bandwidth to fight with you.'

A long pause unfolds. I stare again at the waterfalling snow outside.

'I still want us to be friends. I want you in my life. And Emma's. She adores you.'

'Well, the feeling's mutual, obviously.'

Occasionally, I do reflect on how I would feel if I'd reached this stage of life without having left Josh, or had my daughter. Or even if I'd taken the pill, and then been unable to conceive.

If I'd not listened to the insistence in my heart back then, I would have so many more regrets now. I am sure of that.

I stare at the flames frolicking in the fireplace, trying to focus my thoughts on the stuffed stocking I will hang above the hearth in a few days' time, the icing sugar footprints I will dust on to the stone. The half-eaten carrot and crumpled mince pie foil on a holly-and-ivy plate – all the things Dad kept doing for me after Mum left, so that Christmas stayed magical.

For a moment – I'm not sure why – I think Josh is going to mention the antidote again. But he doesn't.

I gave him his Christmas gift earlier, made him promise not to open it before the big day. I unearthed it in a second-hand bookshop, a rare book for a rare person – a signed first-edition copy of *The Remains of the Day*. It cost even more than what I spent on Oliver this year, but I couldn't resist.

I know it probably wasn't fully appropriate. But, when it comes to Josh, I do have a tendency to forget myself. Which is probably why I hand-drew him a Christmas card, too. A penguin on a snowscape, in a bright red woollen hat and scarf, gazing hopefully up at the stars.

57.

Josh

June 2011

Darren summons me to his place. I try to pretend I'm busy, but then Giles turns up at my flat and practically headlocks me over there.

In Darren's kitchen, I attempt to avoid the discussion I know they want to have by engaging Darren's youngest, Blake, in a long and involved conversation about his Xbox. Unsurprisingly, though, sixteen-year-olds have better things to do with their weekends than explain gaming to Luddites, so he escapes at the earliest opportunity.

Darren's phone buzzes with a message. He glances at it, smiles softly. 'Last exam for Raffy yesterday. Three years down, two to go.'

His oldest boy is at uni in London, studying to be a cosmetic dentist. This kind of blows my mind, given that I first met his parents two years before he was born, and I'm pretty sure his first word was *bum*.

'Just wish that one would sort himself out.' Darren tips his head in the direction of Blake's bedroom. 'I keep trying to tell him, playing Xbox isn't a career plan.'

'Is for some people,' Giles mumbles, through a mouthful of Monster Munch. 'They have tournaments now.'

I feel a flex of guilt for chatting to Blake just now – and, let's be honest, for much of the past sixteen years – about exactly that. Still, I continue to find myself weirdly rapt by these vicissitudes of parenting. Even the stuff my friends tell me is hard, boring, challenging. I envy, oddly, everything.

You always want what you can't have, I guess.

'So, that's it?' Darren says to me, after tapping out a quick message to Raffy. 'You're officially divorced?'

I nod. 'Solicitor sent through the decree absolute last week.'

In a nice little fuck-you from the universe, my divorce certificate came through a decade to the day that Rachel walked out. Ten whole years without her. Ten years of living a life that, sometimes, I struggle to recognise.

'Sorry, mate,' Darren says, putting his phone away. 'But maybe this is what you've needed. Closure. Absolutely zero chance of you ever reuniting.'

'Great, cheers,' I say, offering him a slightly piqued thumbs-up.

Darren and Giles exchange a silent glance.

'What?' I say, a little more bluntly than I intended.

'You should try to see this as a fresh start.'

'Yep. Look to the future, pull yourself together and stop pining after Rachel,' Giles chips in.

I wish it were that easy. Last month, walking past Pizza Hut, I happened to look up and see Rachel, Oliver and seven-year-old Emma at a table in the window. They were the perfect picture of a happy, messy family, all crayons and sticky fingers, half-finished refills of Coke, plates piled with abandoned crusts. Emma was giggling at something Oliver was saying, her whole body tilted sideways in the breeze of his quick wit.

I just stood next to a bin graffitied with expletives and watched them all for a few seconds, my heart racing and aching.

'Define pine,' I demand, by way of deflection.

Giles clutches his chest, starts to speak in a pitched-up voice.

I smile despite myself, hold up a hand. 'Forget I asked.'

I haven't ever told them what Oliver said to me, the first time we met. It would only get back to Rachel, and make me look bitter.

I think about Wilf. I wonder if he's started to slowly lose himself over the years too. If he sometimes looks around and can't believe he ended up living in Spain, playing poker to make ends meet. How he feels about time passing, seeing an unchanging face staring back at him in the mirror. If he ever fears the future, or gets the sense he's being left behind. If he stalks his old friends online, marvelling at the fact that their kids are doing things like learning how to veneer teeth, while he's stuck in the early noughties, attempting to style it out.

I've tried calling him a few times since my visit to Spain. But the only number I've got for him always comes up as out of service.

It still troubles me deeply that Darren and Giles have long-assumed Wilf simply upped and left us all, too selfish to provide so much as a functioning phone number. They've stopped discussing how they think he's doing these days, so I can only conclude they no longer care.

'You should try to see this divorce as a positive,' Darren says. 'The start of a new chapter. You need to look forward. You're not still considering that antidote idea, are you?'

I shake my head.

'Good,' says Giles. 'I mean, reversing it could put you right back to where you started, no?'

I don't respond. I hadn't actually thought of that.

Eventually, I decided against taking things any further with Wilf's ex-colleague Hester. Rachel has made it clear she will never want the second pill. But for some reason I know I'd still find it impossible to hand it over to a third party, no matter how trusted.

That's not to say I haven't spent a fair amount of time trawling the internet, to see if I might be able to track down a cure for what I did to myself. But, predictably, it's thrown up nothing useful. Just clickbait news pieces about the opposite of what I'm looking for, like collagen and retinol, and the occasional dubious-looking article about 'promising tests on mice'.

'I'd make the most of eternal youth if I were you. I mean, take me, for example. I'm probably going to have a heart attack if I don't join a gym, stop eating butter, cut back on—' Giles breaks off to up-end his bag of Monster Munch, shaking the remnants into his mouth.

Across the table, I meet Darren's eye and we share a smile.

'I've started creaking when I stand up,' Giles continues, through his mouthful. 'I need more time to recover between shags. And, last night, I needed to piss twice. *Twice*.'

'You're forty-three.'

'Exactly. Clock's ticking. The girls are going to be *teenagers* in a month. Next thing I know, they'll be off to uni. And then . . .' He trails off and wipes his mouth, seeming dangerously close to becoming emotional.

'You could still have kids,' Darren says to me. 'You could still meet someone. You always wanted a family.'

Giles nods sagely. 'The point is, you've got time. *Infinite* time. You never have to worry about your sperm going stale, or being too old. That's a *gift*, mate. Make the most of it.'

I walk home alone, trying not to dwell too hard on the concept of stale sperm. My route takes me past the takeaway that used to be Sorelli's. Its neon sign glows red and blue in the dark, the smell of grease and deep-fried chicken wafting through the humid air. The night sky has blown pale, skimmed now with creamy clouds.

Still Falling For You

I think back to all the times I sat inside those walls with Rachel, spilling spaghetti sauce on my T-shirt and talking nonsense and trying, always, to make her laugh.

For a while I stand on the opposite pavement, watching teenagers mill around the shop, buckets of chicken in hand. Our laughter, I realise, has been replaced. New kids are here now, carefree and on the cusp of their futures.

And it is this most unlikely of tableaux that makes me think, yes – why keep living in the past? Because I can never take back what I did.

The world has moved on, and Rachel has too. So maybe my friends are right. Maybe, finally, it's time I did the same.

SECTION IV

58.

Josh

June 2012

I have just finished a hot yoga session when one of my classmates runs outside to catch up with me.

I've noticed her before, but have always avoided making eye contact – I mean, it would seem slightly odd to do anything else, in a group environment where you're all semi-naked.

Piles of russet-coloured hair, damp from the shower. Green eyes, a full face of freckles. Mouth fluttering, a beguiling smile.

'So,' she says, resting a slim hand on my arm. 'Are you a fully paid-up member of this wellness wankery, or do you fancy getting a drink?'

We find a quiet corner together in a nearby bar, which is musty, dark and dead. But there is something electric about Andrea. Her green eyes are almost cat-like, winged with dramatic sweeps of eyeliner. She has the kind of laugh that reaches into all four corners of the room. Every third word, a part of her body touches mine.

'Teetotal?' she asks, but not like she's judging, just curious. She's gone for cider; I've stuck to lemonade.

I shake my head. 'Just taking a break.'

'Good for you. Very disciplined. Nothing worse than a vice gone rogue.' Sipping her cider, she makes searing eye contact over the rim of the glass. 'So, tell me, Josh. How old are you?'

For a brief and startling moment I wonder if, somehow, she knows. Or whether my body has finally – incredibly – begun responding to the passing decades while I've been looking the other way. 'Why do you ask?'

She's eyeing me as you might a piece of art you think you like but don't quite get. 'You seem like one of those people who looks an awful lot younger than they are. A kind of ... British Paul Rudd. Plus, I quite fancy flirting with you, so I need to establish what I'm dealing with.'

I laugh for what feels like the first time in a while. And, for once, it isn't forced. I am, unusually, quite up for being flirted with.

And something else feels new, too. The reassurance I draw from how perceptive she is. She reminds me a bit of Rachel in that way. Because, in my experience, enquiring minds also tend to be the most empathetic.

And so I do what I never do, and tell her. Everything. The whole story. The only bits I miss out are Wilf's name, and what it did to my marriage.

Maybe telling her is a test. To see just how into me she is.

'So how old are you, exactly?' she asks, when I'm done. 'Chronologically, I mean.'

'Forty-two, just.'

'Bloody hell. Lucky you.'

'Well. Yes and no.'

For a while, I thought eternal youth might eventually lead me to enjoy birthdays. But if anything the dread of them only ever deepened. Time has turned now into an outgoing tide, from which I have become stranded, a barnacle on a reef.

Andrea tilts her head. 'Why bother with yoga, then? I mean, I assume you don't need to exercise or watch what you eat or panic about blood pressure like the rest of us. Or stress about death or disease or Viagra.' She makes a little whooping sound. 'What a bloody gift that must be.'

I can't help smiling. Andrea told me, on our walk over here, that she's not yet thirty-four. 'Do *you* have to stress about Viagra?'

She smiles back. 'From time to time. Anyway. It must be very liberating.'

'Actually, the yoga's more of a mental thing, really.' I don't tell her I've joined a gym and breathwork class lately, as well. That I've been taking my friends' advice and trying to sort my shit out, focus on the future, stop thinking about Rachel. I've deleted her number from my phone, though this was a token act more than anything else, since of course I can recite it off by heart. I recently quit the needless nicotine too, have cut right back on booze, am getting into cold showers. And I've been spending a fair bit of time in my garden, with my mum. It's been nice, actually, Mum and I tidying and pruning and chatting, planting the flowerbeds over for wildlife. I've even dug a pond, to attract the frogs and newts and bats. It's a form of meditation, I guess. A way to self-improve, attempt to pursue a more peaceful life.

'The never-ageing man,' Andrea muses. 'I could put you in a book.'

The term makes me flinch slightly, but curiosity overrides my discomfort. 'You're a novelist?'

'I am.'

I tell her I'm an author too, ask what type of books she writes.

'Experimental fiction, mostly,' she says. 'Themes of isolation, failure, deception. All the cheery stuff.' She names her latest novel.

'Wait – you're Andrea Bewley?'

'That's me.'

'Wow, you're . . .' Literary royalty, basically. She was shortlisted for the Booker, I think, the year before last. She also wrote *In Spite of Him*, one of my top-ten books of all time. 'I didn't know you lived around here,' I say, feeling more than a little dazzled, and wishing I could take back around ninety per cent of the stuff I've said to her over the past half-hour.

'Divorce. I moved back.'

'Oh,' I say. Then, 'Sorry.'

She shrugs. 'No need. You could congratulate me, if anything. But what about you? Doesn't your wife mind you meeting strange women for drinks?'

'Ex-wife. So, no. Not really.'

She arches an eyebrow, nods down at my wedding ring.

I realise she's ribbing me. 'I'm kind of used to wearing it. It's a bit tragic, I know.'

She agrees with a smile. 'Okay, next question. Do you only go for women in their twenties now you've taken your youth elixir?'

I laugh uncomfortably, shake my head. 'You literally couldn't be more wrong.'

'Oh. Good,' she murmurs, and I feel her gaze ripple into me like a series of tiny tidal waves, one after the other.

59.

Josh

June 2012

We go back to Andrea's place, a flat close to the river. It's not dissimilar to mine, only hers is three storeys high, right up in the eaves. It is romantic in a way I imagine apartments in Paris to be, with creaking floorboards and crooked doorways and twinkling vistas of the skyline from the sloping windows.

'I could have got somewhere bigger, after the divorce,' she says, watching me as I take in the view, then examine her bookshelves – all the literary greats – and the awards gongs on her sideboard, the myriad photos of her grinning with a gang of women I assume to be her girlfriends. 'But I've always dreamed of a writer's garret.'

'Yeah,' I say with a smile, because I know exactly what she means.

She offers me coffee, and I go with her into the kitchen. We face each other as the kettle boils, talking the whole time. But then – as she's measuring out the coffee, and I'm wondering if I should try to say something clever about T.S. Eliot – she says, 'Oh, honestly, fuck this, don't you think?'

She drops the spoon. Coffee granules scatter everywhere. She hooks a finger into my belt, tugs me towards her. Our lips do not so much meet as clamp together, our tongues colliding moments later. She tastes of cream soda, the flavour of the vape she was pulling on the whole way home. She moves closer, pressing me up against the worktop, hand grasping the back of my neck. No mercy, that's Andrea.

After a few moments, she leads me out of the kitchen and into the bedroom. Keeping the lights off, she feels for my T-shirt, pulls it up and over my head. I tease the dress from her shoulders, let it fall in a twist to the floor. She moans a little, breathes out my name. She arches into my hands, her skin shimmer-warm. A groan passes from my mouth to hers. I kiss her harder.

We move on to the bed. Every part of my body is pulsing, straining, roaring with want. I can't wait any longer. I reach for her hips, pull her on top of me.

Afterwards, she pushes the hair from her face, lets out an amusingly satisfied sigh. 'Well, if that was being a cougar, I'll take it.'

I can't stand that word, as it goes, but right now Andrea could sling any kind of ageist slur my way and I probably wouldn't object. So I just smile and shake my head.

It's the novelty, I think. Of actually being with someone who knows the truth. Not feeling like I'm deceiving her somehow, or constantly trying to calculate whether the age gap I've concealed is too much.

'God, you're blushing!' Andrea exclaims, with a nudge to my ribcage.

'It's hot in here, actually. Not sure if you've noticed.' This isn't a lie. It's pretty stuffy up in the eaves, and I am spent now, slick with sweat.

'Don't worry,' she says teasingly. 'I like bashfulness. My husband was an outrageous exhibitionist. Which is actually incredibly boring.'

Out of nowhere, I find myself picturing Lawrence. 'How so?'

'Well. One-man shows usually are, aren't they?' She traces shapes against my skin with a fingertip, making me shiver all over again. 'So, I take it you're sure the pill has worked?'

I slide an arm behind my head. For many years, I was undecided. Hesitancy hovered in my mind like heat haze, the real answer never quite distinct. But recently, all doubt has evaporated entirely. I can see the truth in the mirror, without question – in my supple skin and bright eyes. My still-sharp jawline and stalled stubble, the going-nowhere ridges of my physique. 'For a long time, I wasn't sure. But now? Yeah. I'm pretty certain I haven't aged a day in the past twelve years.'

Andrea talks a lot, but she's good at listening too. So I tell her about the full-body MOTs I've been having again lately – and that, every time, my stats come back exactly the same. Identical, down to the decimal point. The doctors always seem surprised, congratulate me on being in prime physical condition for my age. I'm not sure if they know my history. There's certainly no indication of it on any of the tests. It's not as if the pill has sent my cholesterol skyrocketing, or obliterated my neutrophils, or whatever other bits of my bloodstream they like to skim off and quantify. Detectability-wise, that pill has transpired to be roughly on a par with ricin.

I confess that, for a long time, I was trying to find an antidote.

'An antidote? *Why?*' Andrea looks outraged.

I start to think of Rachel, then resist. 'It's complicated.'

Her smile twitches a little. 'I think I'm going to enjoy figuring out how your brain works, Mr Foster.'

It is the first time in a long while that anyone has referred to me using the future tense. It feels oddly nice. 'Well, if you do, can you let me know?'

She laughs again, shakes her head. 'An antidote. Seriously.'

I shuffle back to get a better look at her, all tumbling red hair and blood-rushed cheeks, cream-smooth outstretched limbs. 'Getting older is a gift. You're going to have to trust me on that.'

'I absolutely will not. But life *is* for living. So why the hell aren't you out there making the most of it?'

I reach up to kiss her. 'This does fall under that category, you know.'

She kisses me back. 'Ooh, that was a test. You're good.'

I scan her emerald eyes, the long lick of her lashes. 'Seriously, eternal youth isn't all it's cracked up to be. I don't know why everyone's chasing it so hard. I'd do anything for a few grey hairs. Or a sense of the future being . . . well, finite, at least.'

She leans down to kiss me again. 'You're weird. But that's lucky for you, as it happens.'

'Why's that?'

She spins me an amused gaze. 'Because that's what I'm into.'

'You're not actually going to put me in a book, are you?' I say, thinking back to her remark from earlier.

She snorts. 'Sorry, my heroes are all morose old men with holes in their socks.'

'I can be morose. And most of my socks have holes.'

'No,' she says thoughtfully. 'You're far too handsome and brooding. I could always pivot into romance, I suppose. Write a rompfest.'

'Please don't. I love your work.'

'Do you?'

'Don't sound so surprised.'

'Men usually object to reading me.'

'I love you,' I say. And then, eyes wide, 'As in, I love—'

'Oh no, let's leave it at that.' She trills a laugh, rolls on to her back. 'Well, this has turned out to be quite the unexpected encounter, Josh, hasn't it?'

60.

Rachel

December 2013

About a fortnight out from Christmas, after picking Emma up from school, I sit alone for a while in our kitchen-diner before Oliver gets home. I'm attempting meditation, ten guided minutes via Ingrid's company's new wellbeing app. She's out in LA promoting it at the moment with Sean, who now works with her as her CTO. They're spending Christmas there, and I will really miss her: each year it's Ingrid who supplies the mistletoe, who insists we do Christmas jumpers and Secret Santa, festive karaoke, rude charades – not to mention destroying us all with the world's most potent eggnog.

Emma comes into the room, still in her uniform, and slides silently on to the stool opposite me. Her hair glimmers gold in the glow of the bulbs I've strung around the room.

I always love this quiet time with her, just the two of us, when things spill softly out of her about school and her friends, small dilemmas and funny things that have happened, ideas for the weekend. And I treasure it, because I know that all too soon she'll be going straight to her bedroom after school and I will be coaxing her to talk to me, having to work far harder to keep track of the person she is becoming.

And perhaps our time together also feels special because she might soon be joined by a sibling. Or is it, in fact, more that she might not? Oliver and I have been trying to conceive for three years now, and, lately, everything we've been throwing at it has been beginning to feel faintly house-of-cards. Hope built with bated breath from fertility vitamins and acupuncture, special tea and scheduled sex, reflexology, guilt trips, tears.

Emma peels the foil thoughtfully from a mince pie. Oliver has a thing about not eating Christmas food before the day itself, but I have a shelf of festive contraband hidden in the larder, which Emma and I enjoy raiding whenever his back is turned.

I shut down the app and take off my reading glasses. 'What's on your mind, sweetheart?' This, I have found, is much more effective than just asking if she's okay, which is far easier for her to shut down by way of a single syllable.

'Did you know that Uncle Josh took a pill to stop him getting older?'

I feel my blood turn to iced water. 'Where did you hear that, darling?'

She bites into the mince pie. 'Dad told me.'

I feel a tiny flare of anger, quick and bright as a struck match. Lawrence cannot have imparted this information by accident. Is he still so bitter about Josh that he would involve his nine-year-old in weaponising his past?

Emma is aware I used to be married to the man she knows as Uncle Josh. But I've never really told her how or why it ended – only that we drifted apart, over time.

We bumped into him in town not long ago. He bought Emma a doughnut, and they chatted about *Harry Potter*, then she grilled him about being an author. I noticed he was no longer wearing his wedding ring, which made me sad and relieved, all at once.

It always seemed to me that Emma and Josh had a special bond. Some of my happiest memories are of Josh making her laugh as a toddler, so hard she'd get the hiccups. He's just one of those people who has a magic touch with kids. I've never doubted he would have been an amazing dad.

Sometimes the guilt swamps me: that I am the reason he never got to do that. That he may *never* get to do it. But then I have to remind myself – as Ingrid would say – that Josh made his choices. Still. The feeling of culpability never quite goes away.

Emma looks up at me. 'Did he, then?' she says, through another mouthful of pastry.

It is hard to believe, sometimes, that Emma is only nine. Because she is already so smart. And we never lie to each other.

I glance for a moment towards the darkened window. There is no point in making this about her father: she wouldn't know why, and it wouldn't be fair. 'Yes,' I say eventually.

'That's so cool,' she says, screwing up the mince pie foil and wiping her mouth.

'What do you think is cool about it?'

'Not ever getting old, or wrinkly,' Emma says.

I smile. 'There's actually nothing bad about getting old, or having wrinkles. It's natural, very normal.' I lean forward. 'I have them. Look.'

What I don't say is that occasionally, fleetingly, of course I fantasise about being twenty-nine again. Firm-bodied and shiny-haired, with skin that looks better under bright light, not worse.

She peers at me. 'No-but-I-mean *really* wrinkly. Like Grandad.'

'Well, I'm sure Grandad would tell you he's proud of his wrinkles.'

'Why, though?'

'Because all of Grandad's wrinkles add up to a million smiles.'

We saw Dad just last night, when he came to ours for tea. He ruffled Emma's hair and called her *poppet*, the way he loves to do.

Oliver asked once if I minded Dad ruffling her hair like that.

'Of course not,' I said, bemused. 'Why would I?'

He just shrugged. 'It tangles so easily,' was all he said.

'Anyway,' I say to Emma, 'taking a pill like the one Uncle Josh took wouldn't just be about appearances, would it? Imagine if everybody decided to take one. The world isn't set up for people to live forever. And if some people took it and some didn't, it might be really hard to know how old someone was, when you met them.'

She nods slowly. 'I don't think I'd like to live forever. Like, loads longer than anyone else.'

'No,' I say carefully, not wanting to veer too closely towards the subject of death. 'Me neither.'

Thankfully, her mind is already wandering. 'Mum, can we finish watching *Home Alone*? Before Oliver gets back.'

There were countless tiny joys I hadn't realised were waiting for me when I first became a mother, and this is just one of them. Snuggling with my daughter beneath a blanket in front of our favourite Christmas film, toes touching, our eyes and smiles meeting at exactly the same moments. I can't wait to watch *The Holiday* with her, too. But she is not quite old enough yet. So, for now, Macaulay will have to do.

I'd been planning to squeeze in a bit more work before dinner. But then I catch sight of my daughter's hopeful face, and check the time. Screw it, it's Christmas. 'Go on, then. Why not.'

61.

Josh

January 2014

Andrea and I are in Valencia, where she's attending a literary festival. I've tagged along for a few of her work events now. Book fairs and signings, trips abroad to meet publishers.

We are eating dinner at an oyster bar. This was Andrea's suggestion – I've never exactly been an oyster kind of guy. Rachel and I tried them once, on one of our semi-ironic Valentine's Day outings, and all I can remember is Rachel crying with laughter as I repeatedly gagged.

It's the kind of place where you have to bray to be heard, all chandeliers and vintage champagne and crustaceans on plates. I wish I could have been brave enough to suggest we give it a swerve in favour of the scruffy tapas joint up the road, which looked far more fun. But Andrea is sophisticated, and this is her trip, at the end of the day. Okay, so oysters aren't my thing. But maybe they could be. And my girlfriend is nothing if not a fan of living life outside your comfort zone.

'Love that people assume you're my toy-boy,' she says, running her foot up my leg beneath the table.

She introduced me this way to her friends, when we first met. She likes pretending we're kind of kinky, teasing me about looking aeons younger than her.

'Very funny,' I say, poker-faced. 'You're thirty-five. We look entirely normal together.'

But, in reality, I enjoy that we can joke about it. I like that she feels comfortable enough to rib me, remind me not to take myself so seriously. I like that joining her for events and dressy dinners and hours-long writing sessions means I have so much less time now to dwell on the future, or how jarring it feels to see a twenty-something when I look in the mirror. I like that I'm constantly thinking about crafting a paragraph she will deem to be perfect, or picking her bunches of snowdrops from the garden, or unearthing old recipes for soups and muffins and soda bread she might enjoy. And I like it when she seeks me out at my desk, kissing and caressing me for what seems like hours before eventually sinking on to me, dress bunched around her waist, fingers raking my skin, face flushed and glimmering as she bites back my name.

She squeezes a lemon segment over an oyster before sipping it from the shell. 'Thought I'd lost you this morning.'

'Had a sudden burst of inspiration at three a.m.'

'Lucky you. What are those like?'

I throw her a sceptical look. She's always complaining of having creative block, yet she's the one selling out literary festivals, not me.

Still. Meeting her appears to have hot-wired my brain, creatively speaking. Maybe Rachel wasn't wrong, all those years ago. Maybe I really did need a muse. For the first time in a long while I've been feeling reinvigorated by writing, pouring words on to the page, unable to stop, as if I'm crafting my debut all over again.

This new novel is different from anything I've written before, though. Genre, subject matter, form. Which feels like a risk, in many ways. Then again, I can probably afford to take one now. The idea I discussed with my publisher a few years back went nowhere; I promised myself I would give it my best shot, but the whole project was canned before I'd even written a word.

'I'd love to read what you've got so far,' Andrea says, sipping her champagne.

To most writers, even a single sentence of feedback from Andrea Bewley would be literary gold. And I include myself in that: since we met, we've spent countless evenings debating narrative convention and technique, voice and characterisation, genre, drive, intention. She is, to be frank, the hottest teacher I've ever had. In fact, it's started to make me question what I ever thought I was doing, masquerading as a college lecturer and imparting what I now know to be my distinct lack of expertise.

Being with her has focused my mind to an entirely new degree. Because I am keen to impress her? Or maybe it's because we are not so different. We both want to write books that other people admire. I find myself talking to her about writing more than anything else, in the hope of absorbing even a smudge of the creative energy that propelled her to the top of the bestseller lists.

That said, I'm not quite ready to share what I've been writing yet.

'It's really just brain vomit right now,' I tell her.

'Mmm, that is a good stage. I do love a good creative puke.' She nods down at the oyster platter. 'Go on, then.'

Gingerly, I take one and raise it to my lips, bypassing the lemon and black pepper, because no amount of garnishing is going to make a dead mollusc taste good. I want to get it over with as quickly as possible. So I tip back my head and down it in one, the way I've read you're supposed to.

Andrea smiles, leans towards me and whispers, 'Swallowing whole is kind of a giveaway, you know.'

'Of what?' My mouth tastes of fish and seawater. Why the hell do people eat this stuff?

'Amateur oyster-eater,' she says, but with a fond smile, as if she thinks it's cute.

I was already feeling faintly self-conscious next to Andrea, in her waft of dark blue silk and vault's worth of silver jewellery. I just packed my usual uniform of plain dark T-shirts, jeans and trainers to come out here. I guess it's my way of trying not to attract attention, to blend in, do my best to avoid eye contact with anyone I don't know.

But, lately, I admit I have been wondering if I need to up my game. To begin dressing more smartly, perhaps learn about things like fine food and opera, watch more films that come with subtitles.

'Hey, I've been thinking.' She is gazing at me now, chin resting on cupped hands. Her red hair drapes in waves down the front of one shoulder. 'Tomorrow, you should get out there and network. I can introduce you to whoever you want.'

I always feel vaguely uncomfortable about being professionally associated with Andrea. I'd hate anyone to think I'm trying to piggyback off her talent. Me, the unknown nobody; her, the literary giant. Andrea always scoffs at this, tells me that everyone networks, that refusing on principle is senseless and short-sighted. And, realistically, I can't disagree. If I'm going to get to where she is, I need to start taking her advice on all this stuff.

That said, I have been wanting to suggest an alternative way to spend some of our free time while we're here.

Google tells me Torrevieja is only a couple of hours away by car, which has made me wonder if we could find the time to try to see Wilf. We could take a trip there together. Hire a convertible, grab coffees, drive the coast road.

But Andrea is still unaware that Wilf was the pill's inventor, and I haven't quite squared yet what I'd say if it came up. So perhaps that's why the suggestion eventually stalls in my throat. Andrea and I have disagreed over Wilf before: she insists I'm too sentimental about him, this friend who purportedly left the country for no reason and abandoned all his friends. She tells me I should cut him off for good.

I both admire her ability to jettison anyone who has crossed her, and deeply fear it.

So, instead of proposing a road trip, I suggest doing something else. Something I've been thinking about for a while.

'Move in with me. When we get home.'

In the eighteen months we've been together, Andrea and I haven't discussed the future much. She's really a here-and-now type of person, which so far has suited me fine.

I did take off my wedding ring just two days after we met, though. This might sound long overdue, especially since Rachel and I were already divorced. But, to me, it was a big deal. I'd never wanted to do that for anyone other than Andrea.

If she's surprised by what I've just suggested, her face doesn't betray even a flicker of it. She lifts her champagne glass, silver jewellery sparking in the candlelight. 'You know I said I'd never live with anyone again.'

True – she has told me this before. She's written entire magazine articles about how badly her divorce burned her. But, if I know one thing about Andrea, it's that she's a risk-taker. So why shouldn't she roll the dice on me, too?

'For the rest of your life?' I say. 'For fifty-plus years, you're not going to live with anyone again?'

She tilts her head. 'What's so radical about that? And more to the point, why are you killing me off in my eighties?'

She's playing for time. 'Is it my age?'

'What?'

'Does the eternal youth thing bother you?'

'No. You know I find it fascinating. The never-ageing man.'

She calls me this occasionally, and it makes me flinch every time.

Andrea leans towards me, tapping a fingernail on the table as if we're resuming the debate we had last night on metafiction – which I lost, obviously. 'I'm actually looking forward to spending a lot of time with you, Josh. Especially if I'm going to get older while you're keeping fresh as a peach. But I just don't want a conventional life. Cohabiting. Marriage. Kids. All that stuff.'

Most of the women in Andrea's novels rail against the patriarchy, any kind of traditional existence. So I already know I'd have to be an idiot to attempt to talk her into any of that.

But the truth is, that isn't what I'm trying to do.

For a long while, I agonised over what Darren and Giles said to me two and a half years ago. *You always wanted a family. You've got time. Infinite time.*

In theory, that remains true. But I think, for me, the dream of fatherhood is probably over now. Maybe because my brain is still wired to believe that, even for someone with a limitless lifespan, the window for having kids – maybe twenty-five years or so – eventually closes. I'm just not sure humans are supposed to hanker after procreation indefinitely.

Anyway. The only girl I ever really wanted to do that with is gone.

But can't living with Andrea just be about wanting more of each other? My flat feels empty whenever I'm in it without the company of her rolling laugh, her salty wit. Time seems to tick by a little slower. I love listening to her chatting to friends as she cooks, humming as she emerges from the shower, even arguing with her agent over the phone. On the nights we spend apart, I miss kissing her and craving her, the take-charge way she fucks.

She rests her feline eyes against me now, affects a small pout. 'Were you expecting an answer straight away?'

'Well, maybe a holding response, at least.'

A smile feathers her lips. 'All right. I'll consider it. But in the meantime I think we should go and find out if oysters really are an aphrodisiac.'

'You must already know the answer to that.'

She knocks back the last of her champagne, cool as you like, then brushes my ankle with the toe of her kitten heel, raises a hand for the waiter. 'Why do you think I suggested it?'

62.

Rachel

May 2014

Oliver and I have just bought our first house together, and we moved in yesterday. He had to go straight back to work this morning, so my dad has come over to help unpack boxes.

When we break for tea in the kitchen, he tells me he bumped into Josh the other day. 'He was with a young woman. Red hair. She's a famous writer, apparently.'

'Andrea,' I say, as I de-foil a chocolate teacake. I don't mention that when I tried to read a sample of Andrea's work on Amazon it was so convoluted I couldn't get more than a few paragraphs in.

Eight years my junior, Andrea is beautiful in an immeasurably elegant way. Pale-limbed, red-haired perfection. I didn't instantly warm to her, though. She speaks over people a fair bit, and has one of those laughs that makes other people turn and stare, and not necessarily in an appreciative way. Oliver, of course, thinks the sun shines out of her arse, though I'm pretty sure that's only because he's relieved to see the cold, hard evidence that Josh has moved on.

Josh seemed enraptured, the first time I met her. As if he couldn't believe Andrea was his – or he was hers. The smile didn't leave his face the whole night. His eyes tracked her everywhere she went. But I found myself a little afraid to talk to her, partly due to her booming voice, and also because I'd already heard her use several words I didn't understand.

'You don't like her?' Dad says.

I sigh, draw a finger along the gleaming granite worktop. Since we moved in, I have been feeling a strange urge to rough this vast, pristine house up a bit, spill some stuff or smear a surface or two, to make it feel lived-in at least.

'When we met, Andrea told me she couldn't imagine anything worse than having kids.'

Dad finishes his biscuit then sets down his tea, begins to unwind the bubble wrap from a picture by his feet. 'Well. That's her prerogative, I suppose.'

'Absolutely. But I had Emma with me at the time.'

'Ah.'

'And afterwards, Emma asked me what Andrea meant, and it opened up a whole conversation about where babies come from, and ... it just really pissed me off. It was a completely inappropriate thing for her to say in front of a child. Three gins or not.'

'Your mother loved a gin,' Dad says thoughtfully. He lifts the picture from its wrapping. It is a painting I did of Emma, laughing into sunlight. 'Oh, yes. This is beautiful.'

I brush a few chocolatey crumbs from my fingers. 'Anyway. I'm in the minority. Everyone else adores her.' I try not to sound too petulant as I say this.

'Even Ingrid?' Dad says with a smile.

I smile back at him, but it stings a bit. Last week, Ingrid announced she's relocating to LA permanently with Sean, at the end of the year. I'm ecstatic for her, and faintly awestruck too, because she built that company pretty much solo, from nothing but hard graft, leaps and risks. But I can't help being terrified as well. Of losing her. Of missing her. Of how it will feel, when there are five thousand miles between us.

I change the subject, try to lift the mood. 'Can you believe Emma's going to be ten next week?'

Dad's eyes warm instantly. 'Not in the least. My little poppet, hitting double figures.'

It is still one of my favourite things, to watch the two of them together. Dad making her dissolve into giggles with tickles and winks. The way she runs full-pelt into his outstretched arms after any time apart. How often she seeks him out, just for a hug. That he still offers to read her stories at bedtime, and she always says yes.

Next week, she will be the age I was when my own mother left. An odd, unimaginable milestone.

'Thank you, Dad,' I say suddenly.

He hesitates, teacup halfway to his mouth. 'For what?'

'Holding it together, when Mum left. For not ever letting me think it was my fault.'

'Actually, you did think that for a while, as I recall.' He frowns. 'You asked me, once.'

'Did I? I don't remember.'

'Ah. Well, that's a relief. Must have done something right, then.' He clears his throat. 'Anyway, my darling. It really isn't a thank-you thing.'

63.

Josh

July 2016

On Andrea's thirty-eighth birthday, we go to a new bar to celebrate. It's one of those subterranean speakeasies, all velvet and no lighting and cocktails that taste even grimmer than they sound. I feel out of place, even as a supposed twenty-something.

When I get there – late, because my college class overran – Andrea is deep in conversation with Polly. But Rachel is alone, looking at her phone, so I take a seat next to her.

I glance at her martini glass, which is garnished with a pickle. Ever since Giles let slip that she and Oliver have been trying to conceive, I occasionally find myself checking to see if she's drinking, wondering if today might be the day she tells me she's pregnant again.

Misinterpreting my curiosity, she nudges the glass towards me. 'Try it. It's actually not bad.'

'No, thanks. Think I'll stick with the most disgusting drink I've ever had.'

She lets out a laugh, though it's almost lost to the noise of the bar. 'What's in it?'

'Headline ingredients are chocolate and absinthe.'

'That sounds dangerous.' Her brown eyes meet mine, just for a moment, then she looks away, sips the pickle-martini. 'Hey, do you have any book news for me?'

I've told her before that I've been working on something.

But she doesn't know yet that I have something pretty big to share with her.

I finished writing my latest novel just a couple of weeks ago, and it's been out on submission less than twenty-four hours. And now – after being apathetic for so much of my career that I've sometimes wondered if he's died without anyone telling me – my agent, Melvin, has apparently pulled off the impossible. The news came in this afternoon, via a rare phone call: a sizeable pre-empt has landed, from one of the Big Five publishers.

When he told me, I dropped to the floor in shock and promptly hung up. Then I lay flat on my back and stared at the ceiling.

Bloody hell.

It's already earned me more than my first five novels put together. It is, as my mum would say, *silly money*.

Rachel covers her mouth when I tell her. 'Oh, my God. Josh, that's—'

'I know.' I can't stop the smile from breaking over my face. 'I know. It's mad.'

'It's better than mad. It's bloody brilliant.' She puts her arms around me, buries her face in my neck. She's had a drink, and maybe she wouldn't be hugging me like this if Oliver were here. He's not, though: he's in London at some entrepreneurs' networking back-slapping thing, which means for once I can chat to Rachel without feeling pick-axed by his gaze.

Anyway, tonight, I don't care. Rachel was there through so many of my writing ups and downs. She helped get me where I am tonight, and I want to share this with her.

We hug for a couple of moments. Her gold hair is spilling through my fingers. It's still long enough to reach halfway down her back, has barely changed since she was twenty.

Suddenly, my skin senses that someone is watching us,

from across the room. And I know without having to look that it is Andrea.

Releasing me, Rachel springs to her feet, then dashes to the bar, orders three bottles of champagne. 'We are celebrating, *now*.'

Which is when Andrea comes over to ask what's going on, and I tell her, and she just stares at me, like, *What the fuck?*

We get back to my flat at around midnight. After four years of dating, Andrea and I still haven't moved in together. Eventually I stopped asking, and tried to appreciate what Andrea kept saying about the flexibility of having two separate places, especially where writing is concerned. She spends much of her working day wandering about making coffee and talking to herself and getting her beta readers on the phone. I am more of a headphones-on, do-not-disturb kind of guy. So it is probably better, on balance, that we do have two flats, albeit they are in different parts of town.

I switch on the overhead light, just in case Andrea has been thinking I'll try to incognito my way out of this.

'I'm sorry,' I say, before she can speak. 'That isn't how tonight was supposed to go.'

'The biggest moment of your career, and you tell Rachel – no, in fact, you let *her* tell the entire bar – before you tell me. I mean, it was actually quite impressive, as a territory move. Announcing your news as if it was her own.'

I swallow. My mouth still tastes of that dodgy cocktail, a horrible combination of absinthe and the kind of non-chocolate you find in health food shops.

It is unforgivable, I know. Aside from anything else, I have no doubt that Andrea's influence on my writing has helped get me to this point. And she's my girlfriend, for God's sake. I owed her at least the basic courtesy of sharing the news with her first.

'Has she read it?'

I shake my head, then try to take her hand, light sparking against my watch as I do so. To this day, Andrea has no idea it was my thirtieth gift from Rachel. Thankfully, though, she's never asked.

But she warns me off trying to touch her with a headshake. Her red hair is wild and loose now, making flames around her face. She takes a step back, folds her arms.

'I assume you're aware she still has feelings for you?'

At this, I stiffen. I have sensed coolness occasionally, between Rachel and Andrea since we've been together. But I'd assumed that was normal in these situations. Like the standoff I share with Oliver, who will never not be itching to *schadenfreude* me, the very first chance he gets.

But Andrea hasn't ever intimated that she's been thinking this.

'Andrea, she doesn't. She's with Oliver.'

'Mmm. He wasn't there tonight, though, was he, while she was all over you?'

I could respond by saying Rachel's just tactile, which she is. But that would amount to a shifty attempt to invalidate Andrea's feelings, and I don't want to do that. So I try to tell her what I think must be the truth.

'Rachel always wanted this for me. And she'd had a couple of drinks, and honestly – I think she just forgot herself. But there was nothing in it. I swear.'

Andrea tilts her head. Spots of pink have erupted on her pale cheeks, her green eyes turned almost acidic. 'You didn't speak up, though. You're not the innocent party here, Josh.'

I swallow, chastened. 'You're right. I'm sorry. I know how shitty that must have made you feel.'

'You made a beeline for Rachel before you'd even said hello to me.'

I shake my head. 'Only because you were talking to Polly, and Rachel was on her own. I didn't think. I wasn't thinking, the whole time. My mind was all over the place. Today's been pretty nuts. Please, I love you. If I could reverse tonight and do it all over again, I would. This wasn't how it was supposed to go at all.'

For a couple of moments she just gazes at me. 'Does it ever occur to you to wonder why you spend so much time regretting the choices you make?'

Touché. But I don't clap back. She has every right to be annoyed.

Andrea doesn't say anything else after that. She just walks out of the living room and leaves me standing in the middle of it, feeling elated and completely crushed, all at the same time.

I don't end up following her to bed. Partly because my phone doesn't stop buzzing with texts and emails and social media notifications. Offers from foreign publishers have started to land now. Melvin must be ninety per cent caffeine at this point, putting in the shift of his life. He's probably communicated with me more during the past twelve hours than he has over the course of nearly three decades.

I decide to compose a message to Wilf. I want to tell him my news, even though he never got back in touch, following my visit to Spain. I've fallen down a bit of a YouTube rabbit hole of late, watching videos of Wilf crushing his opponents in various poker tournaments. It's been hard to believe, sometimes, that I've had to turn to social media to keep up with what he's doing, these days.

But in the end I have no idea what to say, really. So I decide to junk my message to him. He might not welcome a cloud-nine update from me when his own career has ended up being poker or nothing. I think I have long known, deep down, that our friendship is over. And maybe it's time for me to accept it.

64.

Rachel

May 2017

'Well, poppet,' Dad says to Emma from his hospital bed. 'How does it feel to be thirteen?'

Perched next to him, she smiles and shrugs. 'Same as twelve, actually, Grandad.'

'I don't believe that for a minute. You could get a part-time job now. Help your mum out with the bills.' He throws me a wink.

She scrunches her nose. 'What? Grandad, I have *school*.'

I laugh as I get out my phone. 'Right. Shall we have a photo? Birthday selfie?'

Emma lifts up her own phone. 'Can I go and FaceTime Freya first? There's no signal in here.'

'All right. Just don't wander off too far, okay? This place is a rabbit warren.'

Dad and I watch my daughter leave to video-call her best friend, birthday trainers squeaking along the freshly mopped floor of the ward, long hair swinging between her shoulder blades.

'She's stopped letting me take pictures of her now,' I say to Dad.

'You were the same at her age, as I recall.'

'So, what did you do?'

His smile twinkles. 'I never stopped asking.'

I smile back at him, my ninety-three-year-old father, propped up on a stack of pillows. He looks a little pale, but, mercifully, much brighter than when I arrived. 'Hey,' I whisper, grasping his hand. 'Are you starting to feel better now?'

'Ah, it was all just a fuss about nothing.' He glances over to the doorway, at which his eyes crinkle with delight. 'Here he is. The man of the hour.'

It's Josh. He's carrying two coffees, a carrier bag swinging from one wrist.

Heart pinching, I swallow hard, stare down at the lino floor.

'You're looking perkier,' he says to Dad, approaching the bed.

Dad had a fall last night, at somewhere close to midnight. Oliver and I were out, my phone buried deep in my handbag. So, in a panic, Dad called the only other number he knew off the top of his head that didn't involve bothering the emergency services. Josh raced over there, bothered the emergency services straight away and sat with Dad till the ambulance came.

An hour or so later, I checked my phone to find half a dozen missed calls and a calm voicemail from Josh, telling me what had happened. But his attempt at reassurance could never have stemmed my panic, or guilt. How could I have been so careless? What if Josh hadn't picked up?

Josh passes me a coffee. 'Thought you might need caffeinating,' he says, with the softest of winks.

I want to weep at his kindness. 'Thank you,' I manage.

Josh takes a seat on the other side of Dad's bed. His gaze meets mine, for just a moment, but the tug of it feels so strong, I have to turn my face away.

He clears his throat, passes Dad the carrier bag. 'I bought you a paper. And some grapes.'

'Do people still bring grapes to hospitals?' I wonder out loud as Dad's thanking him.

Josh catches my eye and smiles. 'Apparently.'

'No, I didn't mean . . . Sorry, I meant . . .'

Josh just beams as I continue to gabble.

I take a breath, shut my eyes for a moment, suppress a laugh. 'I meant, *thank you*. That was really sweet.'

Dad pops a grape in his mouth. 'Gosh, haven't had a grape in a while. Lovely.'

Across the bed, Josh just raises his eyebrows at me in mock reproach, lips twitching with amusement. I can only raise my coffee cup, conceding defeat.

Dad eats another couple of grapes, then looks between us and lets out a satisfied sigh. 'Maybe I should hit my head more often.'

'Um, they don't generally advise it, Dad.'

'Well, all I can say is that this is nice. Being in the same room with you two again.'

A silence descends. My blood thunders. I can't look at Josh.

Dad gestures with his arms and says, 'Come on. Shall we have that birthday selfie?'

'The birthday girl's MIA. That would just be a hospital selfie.'

'Well, that's what all the cool kids do these days, isn't it? Take pictures of their cannulas and whatnot. Come on, huddle in.'

'Dad, do you really want to remember this moment?'

'Yes,' he says, looking between us again. 'As it happens, I do.'

65.

Rachel

August 2017

My beloved father has died, suddenly in his sleep, at the age of ninety-three.

When I get the call, I am on my way to discuss a commission with a corporate client. Forgetting entirely to cancel the meeting, I somehow manage to pull on to a soot-stained verge beneath a sky grubby with clouds, at the edge of a dual carriageway. Traffic charges past, oblivious and uncaring, shaking the car as I shake too.

I feel utterly and unassailably alone.

I will never again see my darling dad, who held our lives together when my mother left. A beacon of a man who did his utmost to save and protect me. Whose laugh lit me up. Who had time to talk, always. Who taught me, from the day I was born, that some love is unconditional. That some love never wavers.

His sweater is still on the back seat of my car. He left it in here last week, when I drove us out to the country park, and we sat and looked over the lake and ate slices of lemon drizzle cake together.

I turn to grab the sweater now and bury my face in it, the wool cushion-soft against my skin. As I inhale the fading scent of him, breathing in his kindness one last time, a scattering of cake crumbs tumbles into my lap.

I can't stop thinking about Emma. That she will never again get a hug from her grandad, or have him ruffle her hair and call her *poppet*. That they won't ever finish *Jane Eyre* now, or make her favourite hot chocolate together, with marshmallows and squirty cream. My heart cracks in half for her, at the thought of the grief that is so cruelly coming for her too.

I sit without moving as time collapses around me, before eventually, something impels me to switch on the radio. I scroll through to a golden oldies station, one at which Dad would have huffed and said, 'Cheek of it. I'm not dead yet.'

I permit myself a small, disbelieving laugh. 'In My Life' by The Beatles is playing. One of Dad's all-time favourite songs.

'I love you, Dad,' I say, then turn the volume high, close my eyes and let the tears stream.

The ensuing days are a wind tunnel of grief, cold and relentless. Every hour feels as though it is angled uphill. I am barely able to communicate with Oliver. I frequently stand in the shower for so long, the hot water runs out. Oliver has to take over my email account. I have spontaneous sobbing fits and lose the inclination to eat. I cling to Emma constantly, to feel her heartbeat pressed against me. We cry together. I feel her pain even more acutely than I do my own. She asks me questions I cannot answer, about death and grief and heaven.

I spend hours at a time with Polly and Lo, not saying much, just needing to be around my oldest friends. Ingrid calls from LA to say she is abandoning all work commitments and flying back to the UK for the funeral. I'm relieved. I miss her deeply; Bedford hasn't seemed quite the same since she left. I struggle these days to walk past any of our old hangouts and not feel overcome. The Indian we all loved on Tavistock Street, and our favourite dodgy pub – now a posh coffee shop – and our preferred spot of grassy riverbank for drinking M&S tinnies in summer.

Lawrence tells me Emma's been inconsolable around him too, which is probably compounded by the fact that, at the start of the year, he broke up with his girlfriend Bianca. He got together with her not long after we split, so she's been in Emma's life since she was really just a baby. Bianca promised she and Emma would stay in touch, but already she's begun to drift away. I try not to be angry at Lawrence, for letting our daughter down, because I know that is not how it is, really. Life happens. But now, death has happened too, and I can't help feeling worried for my sensitive, deep-thinking child.

After the funeral, once we're back at home in the living room, Oliver hands me a brandy. I'd probably rather toast Dad with port, because that was his favourite. But Oliver's gesture is thoughtful, and I don't want to reject it.

I have been trying not to dwell too hard today on the fact that, over the decade they knew each other, Dad and Oliver never really became close. In later years, this wasn't helped by the fact that Oliver kept talking too loudly at him, as if he was deaf just because he was old, which I could tell infuriated Dad. And Oliver still insisted on calling him Mr Walsh, despite years of pleas from both of us to use his first name.

I haven't yet told Oliver that Dad left his extensive collection of vinyl records to Josh. But nor have I told Josh: those conversations are for another day.

I know Oliver was annoyed when I invited Josh to the funeral. But the truth is, I didn't just *want* Josh there – I needed him. And I knew it was what Dad would have wanted, too.

'Josh looked well,' Oliver says now, still on his feet across the room from me.

Is it possible to tell I am thinking about Josh, just from the expression on my face? Polly always says it is.

'I didn't notice.'

I did, of course. At the start of the service, I saw Josh slip into the very rear pew. Then, just before they brought in the coffin, he caught my eye, and shot me a soft, infinitesimal wink. His way of saying, *I've got you*. And though I was cold, and shivering, I felt a dart of warmth, as if his hand was locking into mine, to help get me through the final goodbye.

Over the past couple of weeks, I've been unable to stop looking at the selfie we took in Bedford Hospital, just a matter of months ago. The three of us, grinning into the camera, arms around each other. An unplanned reunion that had made Dad so happy.

'Rachel . . .' Oliver is surrounded now by shadow, darkness that leaps when he moves. 'I think I'd feel more comfortable if you and Josh stopped seeing each other.'

Perhaps he has discovered the selfie. I've had the idea lately that he might check my phone from time to time. But I have no evidence, just a hunch, so it would seem risky to bring it up.

I never told him about Josh being at the hospital that day, because I didn't much see the point. And the photo was impromptu, my father's suggestion entirely. So I've persuaded myself I have nothing to feel guilty about.

But I know, in reality, that isn't true. A lie of omission is still a lie.

Yet I cannot quite believe it: the words leaving Oliver's mouth, or that he would choose tonight – of all nights – to do this.

I realise now he has probably been waiting to say this to me since the day we met. I tilt the glass in my hand, watching the brandy brighten in the lamplight. 'You don't get to make that call, Oliver.'

He folds his arms, widens his stance. 'No, I'm serious. I'm sick of being made to look like an idiot.'

I keep my voice low, conscious that Emma is in the room directly above us. 'No one's making you look like an idiot.'

His grey eyes are thunderclouds. 'You know, Josh is nearly two decades younger than you now. And I hate to say this, but . . . he looks it.'

Even though I know this is bait for me to take, I flinch as if he's pinched me. 'What's that supposed to mean?'

'I just can't stand the thought of people laughing at you, Rachel.'

Maybe Oliver is right on some level – that Josh and I are approaching the point at which someone might tilt their head as they try to work out how we know each other. *Work colleagues? Cousins? Age-gap siblings?*

I don't feel old, exactly, when I am side by side with Josh. But I cannot deny I feel old*er*, at least.

Still. I am incredulous that Oliver thinks the way to bring me round to his side of the argument is by insulting me. 'Is this seriously what you're doing? You feel insecure, so you decide to try to make me feel that way too?'

'Just saying what I see,' he says, then shrugs and walks out.

On the surface, yes – his insecurity is about Josh. But I worry it is, in fact, some outdated ego-blow related to our inability to conceive. In the three years since we agreed to stop trying, he's certainly been snippier with me: the odd remark about my clothes, impatience if I've forgotten something, raising eyebrows at my choice of TV, music, food on a menu. Tiny shifts in our dynamic, undetectable perhaps to anyone but us. He's been shorter with Lawrence lately, too. I have started to wonder if he resents me for not wanting to exhaust every avenue that might have led us to get pregnant, and for not being keen to explore adoption. For seeming to recover from the disappointment quicker than he did.

Or perhaps he thinks I was never disappointed at all.

66.

Josh

August 2017

I get home late from the funeral, because I met Giles for a drink afterwards, to debrief.

It was weird, attempting to put into words how I felt about Rachel's father dying. The man who treated me like a son from the first day we met. Who never once questioned what I'm sure he probably felt was a fanciful career choice. Who could make me laugh till I sprayed drink out of my nose. Who loved Rachel to her bones. Whose speech at our wedding brought me to tears. Especially when he said that the day Rachel met me was the first time his smile had felt true since her mother walked out.

I saw Lawrence at the service and wake, for the first time in a few years. When our eyes met, he just nodded solemnly. I appreciated this, given Lawrence has a history of trying to get me to punch him.

But that wasn't the weird bit.

I felt Oliver staring at me the whole time I was there, tracking my every move. I studiously avoided looking at him, but, if our gazes had happened to collide, I wouldn't have been surprised to see him draw an invisible knife across his neck.

On the plus side, I had a nice chat with Emma. Well, I say nice. She cornered me next to the egg sandwiches, before firing a series of dry quips at me. Then she said, 'I think Oliver's just jealous, you know.'

'Um, jealous of what?' I said, caught off-guard.

Her bright blue eyes in that moment felt like lasers. 'That you look about half his age.'

Somehow, I managed to laugh. But what I really wanted to do was hug her, the way I used to when she was small, because her face was still pink and puffy from crying.

I don't hug her these days, obviously. Haven't for a few years. She's growing up, has morphed from excitable, expressive kid into a self-contained, considered teenager. But I am pleased we have managed to maintain a decent rapport. I've seen her and Rachel more often in recent years, and Emma seeks me out to chat whenever we find ourselves at the same barbecue or pub. We talk about writing and books, celebrities I've never heard of, people upturning buckets of water over their heads on social media.

Before she walked off, she offered up a clenched fist. Gently, we bumped knuckles, a silent show of friendship.

Back home, when I switch on the hallway light, I'm surprised to see Andrea sitting on the communal stairs. She's wearing her jacket and trainers, red hair knotted on top of her head. At her feet is a stack of packed bags.

I frown. 'Are you booked on another trip?' She's only just back from her last one, a literary festival in Edinburgh.

'The second run of your proofs arrived this morning,' she says in a hollow voice. 'I signed for them.'

My novel, *Graveyard Heart*, is out in six months' time. The first run of bound proofs for pre-publicity was apparently quite in demand, so my publisher produced another one.

It's a love story, unashamedly romantic. A complete departure from anything I've written before. But it also came to me unnervingly easily – almost as though the novel was fully formed in my head, and all I had to do was transcribe it. That first draft felt like the purest, truest thing I'd ever put on a page.

'I read it,' Andrea says.

I've been nervous about this for a while, trying to work up to handing her my laptop or a proof, then backing out at the last moment. Mostly because I think I know exactly what she will say.

She's been supremely patient so far, respecting my privacy, seemingly concluding this is just the way I like to work. But I guess she got tired of waiting.

I swallow. 'Great. What did you think?'

At this, she laughs. But it is not a warm laugh. In fact, it's the kind of sound a person might make just before they whip out a blade and shank you.

'I think you've known for a long time what I would think. In fact, I can see why you've not let me near that bloody manuscript since the day you started writing it. If you were going to publish a book about your ex-wife, the least you could have done was warn me.'

This is the accusation I've been dreading.

'Andrea. It's not about Rachel. I promise.'

'That you're not even surprised I've said that tells me everything I need to know.'

'Andrea, I *swear*—'

'Do you think I'm stupid?'

'Of course not. You're the opposite of stupid.' I crouch down in front of her, try to take her hands. But she shifts away from me.

'Did you imagine I wasn't going to figure it out?'

'Andrea. You have to listen to me. That book isn't about Rachel.'

'God. Even now, you can't admit it. Which means you're either deluded, or a liar. And don't even get me started on going to her father's funeral. And wearing the watch she gave you. And your wedding ring, for nearly a full decade after you broke up. And so on, and so on. Well, good luck trying to win her back, I guess. You know it's actually kind of pathetic?'

Her words hit me like bullets, one after the other. 'Okay. Look. I'm sorry. I know there's boundaries that have been crossed, and I accept that. I get that I've been insensitive at times. But it was never intentional. Hurting you is the last thing I want, Andrea.'

'Is murder still bad if you apologise?'

Assuming this to be rhetorical, I stare miserably down at her packed bags. 'Please don't go.'

Apparently unmoved, she folds her arms. 'Why not?'

'Because. I love you. I don't want to lose you. Because I've felt more comfortable, more myself, with you than I have with anyone in a really long time.'

'Well, I'm afraid I wasn't put on this earth to make you feel *comfortable*, Josh.'

'That isn't what I meant. Could we at least just take a moment and talk about this? Why don't we get some sleep, and go out for breakfast tomorrow? Just the two of us, no phones, and we can talk.'

She gazes at me for a long moment. 'I don't think so.'

'Please just give me a chance to—'

'I'm not in the habit of seeking out public humiliation. And that's what publication of this book will be for me.'

I shut my eyes. 'That's not what I'm trying to do. I swear. I love you, Andrea.'

'So why have you been at pains to stop me reading that manuscript?'

I sense a tiny window – although it is more of a spyhole, really, in a door that already seems firmly closed – to persuade her that *Graveyard Heart* isn't autobiographical. 'It's my first non-crime novel. And you're a celebrated writer. You're Booker-bloody-nominated. I was worried you might hate it.'

'Well, you were right. I do hate it.' She looks at me with narrowed eyes and a faint smile, as if she's trying to work out what she ever saw in me. As if she's finally realised how out of my league she really is. 'In fact, I've never read anything I've loathed more.'

This hits me harder than even I was expecting. It takes me a while to find my voice, the way it does when you've been winded. 'Well, I'm gutted about that. Obviously. I was really hoping you'd love it. I was hoping . . . you'd be proud.'

She doesn't say anything else. Just picks up her bags, two in each hand, and gets to her feet. Pushes past me, hauls the whole lot out on to the doorstep.

I just stay where I am on the floor, shaking my head, knowing – because I know Andrea – that I don't stand a chance of saving this.

A few seconds later, I hear her sports car start up. She revs it pointedly once, twice. And then she is gone.

67.

Rachel

October 2017

'This is *so* about you,' Ingrid says, waggling her proof of *Graveyard Heart* at me. She is between meetings in LA, swigging alternately from a coffee and something green as we FaceTime.

Ingrid seems to glow a little harder every time I see her, though I guess that's unsurprising, given she now has the wellness world on speed-dial, adds spirulina to everything and claims to have regular facials that involve being rubbed very firmly with some kind of placenta. In contrast, Polly and I are on the sofa at her place, where we've been watching *La La Land* and mainlining chunks of shop-bought rocky road by the fistful, straight from the tub.

I have lost count of the number of people now who have confidently informed me that I am the love interest in *Graveyard Heart*. But I've never asked Josh – the book's actual author – if it's true. And nor will I. The way I see it, he deserves his creative privacy.

Ingrid starts reading from the back cover. '*A love story to define a generation.*'

I roll my eyes, although I am smiling, because I can never be annoyed with Ingrid. I miss her too much. Not that it's hard to find her, these days, if I need a quick fix of her. She's forever popping up on TV, and in papers and magazines, has featured in countless rising star lists, presented her own TED talk, appeared on numerous podcasts. Her app has hundreds of thousands of subscribers now, and the company recently hit a multi-million-dollar valuation. I am infinitely proud of her, my brilliant, fearless friend.

'Has Oliver read it?' Ingrid asks, flipping through the proof again.

'Oliver doesn't read fiction.'

Next to me, Polly pops another rocky road and says, 'What does he read?'

I try to think. 'Cereal packets? Instruction manuals?'

Ingrid suppresses a smile. 'Mmm. He definitely won't get this, then.'

No. He probably wouldn't.

I read it on the very first day the bound proof landed on my doormat, though I could only get through it in short bursts, and kept having to put it down, because I genuinely feared my heart might give out. When I was done, I felt exhausted – but in a good way – from the two-hundred-plus pages of emotional torment.

Over the screen, a pause unfolds.

'What?' I say, feeling a thump of disquiet in my belly as I look between my friends.

Polly lets out a breath. 'Andrea dumped Josh. After reading *Graveyard Heart*.'

'What? Are you serious?'

'She thinks it was about you,' Ingrid says.

Fiercely, I shake my head. 'Josh doesn't do that. Write about real people, or situations. He wouldn't.'

Ingrid shrugs. 'Well, she was pissed off enough to ditch him.'

'When was this?'

'Few weeks ago.'

'Shit. Is Josh okay?'

Polly tips her head back and forth. 'There's so much going

on for him right now, I don't think he's had much of a chance to feel sad about it.'

'He's talking about a launch,' Ingrid says casually. 'Will you go?'

I frown. 'I'd like to, but . . .'

'But what?'

'But Oliver.'

68.

Josh

February 2018

As I make my speech at the standing-room-only launch of *Graveyard Heart*, I wonder how many of the audience are looking at me through the lens of my being Andrea Bewley's ex. Or if any of them are wondering how old I actually am.

So far, I've still told only my friends and family about the pill. But everyone I work with will soon have to know. I assume they've been too polite to ask until now. Or maybe they think I'm just really into fillers. But at least a handful of them – and possibly the few loyal readers I have – must be wondering why this supposed forty-seven-year-old doesn't look a day over twenty-nine.

I've been worrying, constantly, about the world discovering my secret. I panic in interviews about slipping up, getting my birth decade wrong. Saying something that doesn't quite add up, to a journalist who's on the ball enough to notice.

I have had minor concerns, too, that raising my head above the public parapet might reignite the interest of the lunatics who kept breaking into my flat before. I've been quite enjoying the feeling of Big Pharma not being on my back. And I don't want any renewed attention swinging Wilf's way, either.

★ ★ ★

The afternoon after the launch, Mum and I make a trip to Dad's headstone. We sit wrapped up on a bench beneath an aluminium sky, next to a bare-boned silver birch. I've filled a flask with hot chocolate, and we pass it back and forth.

'I half-thought we might see Andrea last night,' Mum says, after a while.

Six months have passed since Andrea left. I've not heard a thing from her, and she's blocked my number. It's as though I never even existed. 'No, that's well and truly over.'

'And no Rachel?'

I shake my head and let out a breath, watch it turn to mist. The graveyard is deserted, the ground rock-solid with cold.

The last time I saw Rachel, she arrived on my doorstep a few days after her dad's funeral with a box of his old vinyls, and informed me she thought we probably shouldn't speak again. I knew it had to be related to the way Oliver had been looking at me during the wake, as if he was waiting for a good window to slip something lethal into my G&T.

Still. I wanted to ask why. I wanted to talk to her about Andrea. I wanted to sit on the sofa together and go through those old records and reminisce about her dad.

It was unfortunate, I suppose, that I had my top off at the time. I'd been doing yoga in the living room, hadn't thought to retrieve a T-shirt.

'Was it about her, then?' Mum asks me now.

'Was what about who?'

'*Graveyard Heart*. About Rachel.'

'What? No. Why does everyone keep asking me that? I told you, I don't base my books on real people.'

At this point, amazingly, she starts trying to talk me through the concept of dating apps. She rummages around in her bag, produces a scrap of paper, holds it at arm's length. 'Plenty. Of. Fish. Quite clever, isn't it?'

I know Mum was sad for a long time, after Rachel and I split. But it's coming up for seventeen years now. So I guess the pain of our parting has faded slightly, for her.

'Is it?' I smile faintly. 'Look, dating apps are no place for people like me.'

She looks outraged on my behalf. 'Why aren't they?'

'Because I look nearly two decades younger than I actually am.'

'Never stopped Mick Jagger.'

'Mick Jagger's in his seventies. What's he got to do with anything?'

'You're very peculiar sometimes. Eternal youth is what everyone dreams of. Take it from an oldie. Imagine if I could rewind to being twenty-nine. Wonderful,' she says, with a wistful sigh.

As she passes back the flask, I can't help noticing the liver spots on her hands. The way they quiver now, ever so slightly. How she keeps clearing her throat, as if the years have somehow lodged there.

'Why don't you try dating someone in their fifties?' The edges of Mum's eyes crease up with affection. 'You're such a catch, darling. I'm sure there would be ladies queueing up to—'

I raise a hand. 'Can we not.' I appreciate the sentiment, but I am very keen never again to hear my own mother describe me as a *catch*.

Mum looks crestfallen, so I attempt to explain. 'I look as though I should be dating twenty-somethings. But in reality, yes – I should be with someone closer to fifty. Even you must understand how messed up that is.'

Navigating this stuff is only becoming more challenging as the years go by. Because the truth is, just as sleeping with a twenty-something would feel too weird these days, so would undressing someone of my own chronological age. I'd find the physical disparity too hard to get over. Nor could I bear to think of people assuming that was my particular kink.

And this was always Rachel's big fear. She refused to accept that I wouldn't eventually start to think of her that way. But, with us, it was different. I knew her too intimately. She was wrong, when she concluded I'd one day become uncomfortable with being married to her.

Her next big birthday will be fifty. But I have never thought of her as anything other than the girl I fell in love with.

69.

Rachel

June 2020

On the night I turn fifty, I am taken aback to see Josh's name flash up on my phone.

It's getting on for three years now since the day I went to his flat after my father's funeral, to tell him we should probably stop seeing each other. When he answered the door with his top off, I felt my breath break to pieces in my chest. In that moment, it took everything I had not to step forward and try to kiss him. The feeling was so strong, I knew my entire world depended on me staying rooted to that doorstep.

'Come in,' he said.

'I can't.'

A silence followed. It was crushingly loud.

'He's making you choose,' he said eventually.

I bit down on the insides of my cheeks, so hard I tasted blood. 'Thank you for coming to the funeral. I really do appreciate it.'

He pinched the bridge of his nose between finger and thumb. 'You don't have to speak to me like I'm your half-cousin twice-removed.'

'Oliver and I—' I began, then broke off.

'Oliver and you what?'

'We're a family,' was all I said.

I've encountered Josh maybe once every six months since then. But on each occasion he's averted his gaze, kept his distance, barely looked in my direction. And, each time, the pain has been like nothing I've ever known. But I've had something to prove to Oliver. Or maybe it's more that I've had something to prove to myself.

Now, though, I dash into the garden to take his call. The air buckles with humidity, a simmer of summer thunder.

'Hey,' he says tentatively. 'Just wanted to say ... happy fiftieth.'

I am not about to give him a hard time for calling. I'm just excited to hear from him. 'Happy fiftieth,' I whisper back.

'How are you celebrating?'

'A little party for three. Emma's been working on it for weeks. She's bought banners and balloons and stuff. There's a piñata and a playlist. It's all very sweet.'

I don't tell him, obviously, that I was wondering earlier what he and I might have been doing together, on our fiftieth birthday in another life. My mind wanders in this way occasionally, but I try to put it down to nostalgic curiosity, nothing more.

Maybe I'm feeling particularly emotional because Oliver and I had our first online therapy session last night, a very odd precursor to a fiftieth birthday. It had been Oliver's suggestion, which made it even more infuriating and baffling when he refused to open up to the therapist (though not before he'd laid into Josh, and – inexplicably – Ingrid), then informed me once we'd logged off that he'd felt very uncomfortable, baring his soul to a stranger. That he thought the therapist's questions had been almost voyeuristically intrusive.

Music is pumping from the living room. Mungo Jerry, 'In The Summertime'. The single which was, according to my thoughtful daughter, number one on the day I was born.

'Well. I should let you get back to it,' Josh says, perhaps misinterpreting my pause.

'No, wait,' I say, heart in my throat. 'I need a break. I've been dancing to K-pop. I'm not lithe and fit like you, remember?'

I hear him smile. 'All right. How's life, Rach?'

I fill him in, tell him Oliver's winding down to early retirement, that next year Emma will be applying to study law at Oxford. He updates me on the latest with *Graveyard Heart*, the stratospheric sales and film option, the fast-flowing foreign rights deals.

'I always knew you'd make it,' I say.

He laughs softly. 'Ah, well. At least one of us did, then.'

'I don't think I ever told you how much I adored it. *Graveyard Heart*. You should have been writing love stories all along.'

On the other end of the line, a lengthy silence.

I take a breath. 'I'm really sorry we couldn't stay in touch. I think about you a lot. It's just been difficult. With Oliver.' Unexpectedly, a tear breaks free, speeds down my cheek. 'I know I probably navigated that all wrong.'

'No, look, hey,' he says softly. 'You don't owe me any explanations, Rach.'

Suddenly, I hear Emma from inside the house, shouting, 'Mum! We're doing the cake! Mum!'

'I should go. Thank you for calling.'

'Thank you for picking up.'

'I could never see your name and not.'

A breath of hesitation, as if he wants to say something else. But then the screen goes dark.

70.

Rachel

August 2022

During the summer following Emma's A-levels, Lawrence takes her on holiday to Turks and Caicos, where he informs her, off the back of one too many rum punches, that he and I never stood a chance when we were together, because I was still in love with Josh.

I doubt he does this out of spite; we are long past pettiness, I think. Perhaps these are even his true feelings, and the rum punch just brought them out.

A few hours after she gets home, Emma finds me upstairs, prone on the carpet in my bedroom, doing a poor impression of somebody attempting yoga. Ingrid sent me a link to a teacher she rates on YouTube, but I'm struggling.

It's at moments like these that I occasionally fantasise about having taken that pill, so at the very least I might be able to perform basic flexibility exercises without feeling like I need a shot of WD-40 first.

Emma perches on the edge of my bed. She's wearing her school leaver's sweatshirt and a pair of faded leggings. Her blonde hair, made several shades lighter by Caribbean sun, is pulled into a long plait.

'Mum, did you dump Dad because you were still in love with Josh?'

A jarring feeling in my chest. I sit up, back creaking. Lawrence's and my official line, when it comes to our daughter, has always been the truth – that we drifted apart.

'No. Who told you that?'

Emma repeats what Lawrence said. She looks bruised, and I feel the ache of it pass to me. Bloody Lawrence, always putting his foot in it. How he got to be CEO of a FTSE 100 company without ending up in jail for insider trading, I will never know.

'I'm so sorry Dad said that to you, sweetie. But he's wrong. He and I split up because we weren't working. It was nothing to do with Josh.' I kneel in front of her and take her holiday-brown hands in mine. They remind me, fleetingly, of summers past, of ice creams and sandpits and dancing through water fountains.

She nods thoughtfully. 'I read *Graveyard Heart* on the plane.'

I swallow. 'What did you think?'

'I think Josh wishes you'd never broken up.'

I feel my stomach roll over as she holds my gaze.

'What about you?' Emma says.

'What about me?'

'Do you wish you'd never broken up?'

'*No.* Because then I wouldn't have you. I wouldn't swap the last eighteen years for anything, darling.' I'm surprised, as I tell her this, that a sentence can be truer than anything I've ever said, yet still feel like a lie.

'Do you still love him?'

I meet her lagoon-blue eyes, feeling my breath buckle.

'God, you do.'

'It's complicated,' I whisper.

A few moments pass.

'And sad,' she says eventually.

'Yes,' I say, because I only want to be honest with her now.

After that, we just sit together for a while, holding hands in the magnolia hush of my bedroom. The one I used to share with Oliver.

Soon after my father's funeral, Oliver started sleeping in the box room across the landing. He said this was because he knew he snored. But I wondered if it was all related to our struggle to conceive. What it had done to our sex life. The unexpressed resentment, the ego-blow.

All issues we could have discussed in therapy, if Oliver had given it more than two sessions before declaring it to be a waste of time and money. He'd been stiff and uncommunicative throughout, proving he was far more emotionally buttoned-up than I'd ever realised.

I've been wanting to confide in Emma about all this, but now I'm not sure. Might she start to question my entire relationship with Oliver – and perhaps then hers, too?

'I love you, Mum.'

My heart jolts me back to her. 'I love you too.'

71.

Rachel

November 2023

'Rachel?'

I sit up. It is the middle of the night. Darkness is at high tide.

'Josh?'

'I need you.'

'I'm here. I'm here. What's wrong?'

I can tell he is struggling to breathe.

'My mum . . . My mum's—'

'I'm coming. I'm coming to get you.'

At Debbie's house, I make tea, and we take it into the conservatory, where we sit together in the cold without talking much, watching the sun begin to throw light into the sky. Condensation clings to the glass. Outside, the grass is sugared with frost.

'Haven't had any sleep,' Josh says, after a while. 'Fireworks kept popping off.'

I swallow. Last night was bonfire night. 'Same for us.'

How strange it is that, even after thirty-five years, fireworks only ever mean one thing to me: Josh.

From somewhere in the house, I can hear a clock ticking. It feels strangely cruel this morning, the sound of time pushing ruthlessly forward.

Josh has a copy of *Enduring Love* on his lap, the page folded down about halfway through. He tells me he lent it to Debbie a couple of weeks ago. 'It's so weird to think she won't find out how it ends.'

I smile softly. 'She told me once she always has a sneak peek at the last page of whatever book she's reading. So, she probably did know.'

At this, he laughs, despite himself. 'Ah, did she?' He looks across at me. 'Thanks, Rach.'

After that, we just sit and watch the sun climb through a salmon-coloured sky, listening to each other breathe. I can still detect, I think, the faintest scent of Diorissimo, Debbie's signature perfume, worn every day since the seventies. I don't ask Josh if he can smell it too.

'The police wouldn't believe I was Mum's son,' Josh says. 'They kept asking me about next of kin.'

'I'm sorry,' I whisper, reaching out to take his hand. Through the glass roof of the room, a tiny stripe of sunlight alights on our wrists, binding them together.

'I know she was elderly. But when it's someone you love, death's never not a shock.'

'Josh.'

He turns to look at me, seeming somehow to have aged, though I know that is impossible. It is the trauma, I think. It has reverberated through his eyes and skin, even the stark scruff of his stubble. Every cell in his body, colonised now by grief.

'I never stopped loving her, you know,' I say.

Outside, the sun shifts, painting his face momentarily gold. His youth, suddenly, is restored. 'I know,' is all he says.

72.

Josh

November 2023

Rachel comes with me to Mum's funeral. Afterwards, she and I take a walk by the river, tracing Mum's steps along her favourite route for a ramble. It is dark now, the air fringed with frost. But the embankment lights are on, long lines of them looping the length of the river, smearing its surface gold.

We pause at the top of the suspension bridge. Rachel leans on the wrought-iron railing and stares out over the chilly water, sighs deeply. She is wearing her cobalt-coloured scarf, the one her dad gave her when she turned fourteen. Patches of it are shiny now from age, years of repeated touch.

'You did well earlier, by the way,' Rachel says. 'With that woman.'

It was hard to believe, but one of Mum's friends showed up to the service with a copy of my book tucked under her arm. She cornered me at the wake, asked if I'd sign it. *Graveyard Heart*, at my mother's funeral. She'd even brought a Sharpie. The request was so unbelievably batshit, I thought at first she was joking.

'Well,' I say, 'you know what Mum was like. Always shoving Sharpies into my hand. She'd probably have been chuffed.'

Rachel smiles. 'That's an understatement. She was *so* proud of you, Josh.'

I've always felt uncomfortable about things like framing certificates marking smashed sales milestones, or displaying awards, or even copies of my books. So Mum did all the bragging for us both. Half of her living room became a shrine to my career. I was always embarrassed by this, which I regretted, of course, as soon as she was gone.

I take in the shifting river with its wet-mineral scent, the cloak of stars around the shoulders of the sky. We are in the centre of town, but our little patch of it here is peaceful as a lake shore.

'Sometimes I wonder what Emma will say about me, at my funeral.'

I frown, not wanting to dwell too hard on the fact that – road traffic accidents or gas explosions or avalanches aside – I will outlive Rachel.

'I worry, sometimes, that she's so independent because of me and Lawrence. Because we split up when she was so young. Maybe she's *had* to be that way.'

A shot of winter breeze ruffles Rachel's hair. She still wears it long, though she told me earlier that Emma keeps encouraging her to cut it. But she's not quite ready. A bit of grey doesn't bother her, she said, but not feeling like herself when she looked in the mirror would.

I picture Emma as I last encountered her, in Polly's kitchen at Christmas. Self-assured and smart, scalpel-sharp. 'I'm pretty sure Emma wouldn't have become who she is today if you and Lawrence had stayed together. Let's face it: one of you would definitely be doing time for murder by now. And all those prison visits would have put her off a legal career for life.'

She looks amused. 'Would you have come to visit me? If I'd been locked up for throttling Lawrence.'

I laugh. 'Well, sure. You'd have needed someone to smuggle in the Tunnock's Teacakes.'

She smiles. 'God. Haven't had one of those for years. Oliver doesn't like chocolate.'

Wow, I think churlishly, *life with Oliver must be a blast*. A man who dislikes chocolate, relaxing, and – she told me once – any type of pasta. I make a mental note to grab her a box of teacakes next time I'm in a supermarket.

It's the first time I've thought about Oliver in a while. A few summers back, when Rachel and I spoke on the phone for her fiftieth, I remember finding our conversation weirdly hard to get over. I just couldn't stop picturing Rachel's party that night. The laughter, her happiness. The cake and the music. A papier-mâché donkey getting a really hard time. And, in the middle of it all, Rachel, twirling around on the end of Oliver's hand.

'I'm actually not coping very well with Emma being at uni.' The words tumble out of her, and suddenly she seems tearful. 'It's been over a year, but I still miss her. Every day. Do you think that's normal?'

I think of my own mum. How, after I left home, she would act as though Cliff Richard himself were standing on her doorstep, whenever I turned up to see her.

'Yes. I think that's completely normal.'

I wonder if part of the problem might be that Rachel has found herself at home alone with Oliver.

'God, Josh, I'm sorry.' Rachel looks fretful now, bites her lip. 'You don't need to listen to me going on about my empty-nest syndrome. We should be talking about you.'

'Ah, no. Honestly. We've been doing that all day. I'm bored of me.'

'Are you seeing anyone at the moment?'

Usually I can talk about this kind of stuff, even with Rachel. But tonight, for some reason, it just feels too raw. Maybe because all I want to do is go home and be comforted by her, and I know that can never happen.

I shake my head. 'Why does it always come down to this?'

'Sorry.' She sounds stung. 'I just want you to be happy.'

'It's a bit late for that, Rach.' I turn my gaze away, work my jaw. My mouth still tastes unpleasantly of funeral food. Ready-salted crisps, sausage rolls.

I feel her looking at me. 'It's not easy for me either, Josh. I think about you . . . *way* more than I should. I think about the life we could have had, and the things we might be doing now, like . . . going on holiday, and fretting about our pensions, and hanging out with the kids we ended up having, and making each other laugh about stupid things that nobody else would get, and poisoning each other with dodgy microwave meals, right up until our last bloody day on earth. Fish pie gone wrong – it takes us both out when we're in our late nineties, but hey, at least we go together.' She draws a long, shuddering breath. 'You don't think I think about that stuff? Like, *all the time*?'

I am silent. I am stunned.

'And, sometimes, I wonder if I made the right choice. If I should have stayed in your flat, that time you offered me the pill, and taken it.'

My mind whirls back in time. 'I thought you walked out that night because you were angry.'

'No, I walked out because I was *this close* to taking it, Josh.' She lifts her fingers an inch apart.

Her voice is raised, breath hot in the frosted air. I see a couple staring at us as they walk past. The bridge sways slightly with their hurried footsteps. I wonder if they're thinking, *What on earth did that man say to upset his mother so much?*

My heart spins violently, as if it's been struck. 'Is this about Oliver? Aren't you happy?'

And then, because it feels right, because it feels like the only thing to do, I take her hand. The edge of her scarf brushes the inside of my wrist. I feel heat pool in my stomach, my pulse quickening.

She lifts her head. The pool inside me becomes a wave. Suddenly, we are a heartbeat away from leaning in.

But then she shudders out a breath, retracts her hand.

'It's not about him,' she whispers. Her expression is indignant and guilty all at once. 'My regrets have only ever been about you.'

73.

Rachel

November 2023

> I think about all those things too, Rach

> I did want to grow old with you. I just didn't want to be the only one.

> I would never have cared

> Bedpans / dementia / incontinence?

> Fuck that. A lifetime of loving you.

Emma is home from uni for the weekend, so I take her out to lunch.

As soon as the waiter has set down our drinks, she covers my hand with hers, fixing me with powder-blue eyes. 'Mum, I need to talk to you.'

Parental panic rises in my throat. Has something happened at Oxford? Does she need money? Is she unhappy, sick, pregnant?

'What's wrong?'

'I think *you* are. You haven't been yourself for months.

Whenever we talk, you seem sad. You're not the mum I remember.'

I feel relieved and uneasy all at once. 'I'm sorry, sweetheart.'

'No, that's not what . . . I mean, what's wrong?'

'Well, I miss you. It's hard, being home alone.'

'But you're not. Home alone.'

'No, I mean, obviously I have Oliver. But . . . I don't know. It just feels strange without you there.'

'Mum. It's really difficult for me to say this to you, but I think I have to.' Her gaze, suddenly, is stern enough to silence a courtroom.

'Okay.'

'I don't think you love Oliver.'

The clatter of cutlery gets loud in my ears.

'And I feel terrible saying that because Oliver's essentially my stepdad and he's a really good guy, but . . . you know I'm right. I think you're less sad about losing me and more sad about the prospect of being by yourself with Oliver.'

I glance over my shoulder, as if Oliver might at this very moment be seated right behind us with an ear trumpet.

'It's Josh, isn't it?' Emma says gently.

'What is? No,' I say nonsensically.

'Mum. Please be honest with me.'

I hang on to her hand as if she's four years old again and I'm worried about losing her in a crowd. 'I moved on from Josh a *very* long time ago.'

'Yeah, with your head, maybe. But what about your heart?'

I am struggling to know what to say. 'Where is all this coming from?'

'I was in the kitchen getting water last night and a message flashed up on your phone, and I read the preview, because it was three in the morning and I thought it might be important. And it said, *Fuck that. A lifetime of loving you.*'

I feel my neck begin to glow red. 'I'm not having an affair. I promise.'

'I never said you were. I know you wouldn't do that.'

'Josh and I just got a bit emotional, after his mum's funeral.'

We nearly kissed, on that bridge. We could have done. But, right at the last moment, something jolted inside me. *You live with Oliver. You* love *Oliver.*

Then: *Josh is nearly twenty-five years your junior.*

And finally, after too many years of wondering, I felt certainty flow through me, clear and frictionless as water. *I did the right thing. We could never have worked.*

I have been thinking a lot lately about getting older. Maybe because Oliver has five years on me, or perhaps because I can feel my body changing. I have got into the habit of constantly examining my hands, because one of my clients is always telling me – apropos of nothing – that your hands give away your age. Still. Though I'm aware of ageing, I have no interest in fighting it. Yes, my skin is a touch dryer these days, which is probably hormonal, and I pause in front of the mirror most mornings, trying to work out if my hair is growing naturally coarser, or if it's something to do with B vitamins. Whether my crow's feet are down to my time of life, or failing to drink enough water. Everything's a guessing game. I thought I knew my own body after all these years – but now, it seems, each day brings with it another unanswered question. It is unnerving, the not-knowing.

But, as Polly and I like to remind each other, the way we look is only one part of who we are.

'Is this why you never changed your surname when you got divorced?' Emma asks, tearing two more slices from the pizza we're sharing and putting one on my plate.

'Has Oliver said something?'

'No. But I'd imagine it frustrates the hell out of him.'

I smile faintly, take a bite. 'Honestly, it would just feel pointless to change it back now, after all this time.'

'I know you sleep in separate bedrooms. I've known for ages.'

'That was Oliver's idea,' I tell her sadly.

She nods, then hesitates. 'Is this how you want to live the rest of your life? Isn't this just existing?'

I say nothing.

'Oliver isn't your Josh, Mum.'

'Emma,' I say, my emotions threatening to unravel, 'Josh and I can't be together, and I've made my peace with that.'

'Plasma,' she says, out of nowhere.

'Sorry?'

'I've been reading up . . . These old dudes in America keep getting injected with blood plasma from younger people. They did a load of experiments on mice. As in, infusions of young mouse blood in older mice restored their mental capacity.'

I frown. 'That sounds—'

'Horrific. Yeah, I know. But the point is, there are all these old men now, taking part in plasma exchange with teenagers, hoping it might magically restore their youth.'

'And has it?'

'Not yet, but there are clinical trials taking place—'

'What are you saying?'

'I'm saying, surely there's a chance the plasma thing could work both ways. It could restore Josh to the age he's *supposed* to be. Maybe if Josh found someone your age, biologically . . . I mean, God – Oxford's literally the home of cutting-edge research. I could put feelers out, ask around.'

It breaks my heart that this is what she's been spending her time and precious energy thinking about. 'If anything viable came up, I'm sure Josh would know about it,' I tell her gently. 'But honestly? I think he's moved past the point of wanting to reverse what happened. He never talks about it any more.'

Emma sighs, her perfect forehead creasing with a frown. 'But still. You're not happy with Oliver. Not really. He isn't what your heart wants.'

He was once, I think. 'Listen, as you get older—'

'Is this what you'd dream of for me?'

I shut my eyes. *Please don't ask me that*.

'Be honest. Is your relationship with Oliver what you would want for me?'

I can't look at her. I keep my eyes closed. 'Oliver's a good person, Em. He's been in your life since you were three.'

'Yeah, and I'm nineteen now. You don't have to do things for my sake any more.'

I smile as I open my eyes again, because, nineteen or not, she cannot possibly understand that everything I do – *everything* – will always be with her in mind. 'Let's stop talking about me. I want to hear about uni. How are your friends? Have you finished your submission for the moot yet? Do you need anything else for the flat?'

'Mum, please do some soul-searching,' she says, almost talking over me. Her blue eyes are fierce. 'Be brave. I get that it's not easy, but I promise I'll be there for you. Whatever you need.'

74.

Rachel

October 2024

It is not, as it transpires, one event or argument that leads Oliver and me to our eventual end. Rather, our demise resembles a thundercloud slowly fattening, a collection of resentments clinging to cold air, the threat of a final storm only ever moments away.

But for me, perhaps, there is one incident that stands out from the rest.

I come home from delivering a piece of work one afternoon to find Oliver red-faced on the landing, heaving a chest of drawers out of Emma's bedroom. His grey T-shirt is blotched with sweat, and he is struggling for breath.

I put a hand on it, this precious chest that has held so many years of playsuits and vests and little pairs of tights, before the ripped jeans and sequinned tops, the secret diaries. 'What are you doing?'

'Making some extra room.'

'For what?' I say, wondering how much more space Oliver thinks two people need in a house that was already too big when three of us were living in it.

'My golf clubs. The wine. All the shoes and clothes and handbags overflowing from your side of the wardrobe. Your canvases, and painting stuff—'

'You can't just . . . This is Emma's bedroom.' A tiny furnace begins to roar inside me as I regard him, sweating out his repressed emotions all over my daughter's things.

Most of her furniture has vanished now, aside from her bed, which is loaded with boxes. Tessellations of rosy autumn light are gliding over the newly empty walls. Our voices echo where they never did before. Dust motes dance in the void he has created.

I think of Polly and Darren, and how sensitively they approached this, when their boys moved out. Discussing it as a family, packing the old stuff up together. Darren would never have done it behind Polly's back.

'Emma's moving to London next summer,' Oliver says slowly, deliberately. 'She's not coming home, Rachel.'

The burning sensation inside me becomes darker, more intense. Hot coals in my chest. These feelings do come, from time to time. Are they to do with my time of life? Or solely down to Oliver? I've been trying to convince myself it's the former, but now I'm not so sure.

'I was only saying it would have been nice if you had asked.'

He doesn't reply, just turns his back and mutters something under his breath.

I don't quite catch what it is, but it sounds very much like *give me strength*.

After this, it takes me three months to muster the courage to say what is in my heart. What has been in my heart for a long time, I think.

Christmas blurs by, and then it is January, and Oliver and I are still recovering from another whirlwind festive period filled with family logistics and Lawrence being awkward about his plans and invitations to corporate parties and rounds of drinks with neighbours and friends.

We are sitting in the car outside B&Q, waiting for a break in the weather, when I tell Oliver it is over.

Rain is plunging from the sky. Great silver sheets of it, making mist where it lands.

He turns to look at me. But there is no anger, or shock, or even surprise on his face. Instead, there is a resignation I have come to know well.

'I've been unhappy for a while, and I think you are too.'

'Unhappy.' He shakes his head. 'What exactly do you mean by that?'

Two people, I think, *who can no longer be bothered to try*.

He puts both hands on the steering wheel, leaning forward until I wonder if he's about to sound the horn with his face. 'Can't say I'm surprised. I think, in a way . . . I've been half-expecting you to say that to me since the day we met.'

We are quiet for a while. Through the windscreen, I watch the storm spook leaves from the trees, shunting them across the tarmac. The wet sky is the colour of fish skin. There are people rushing past, heads hooded beneath umbrellas.

'Are you going back to him?'

'Who?' I say, thinking for a moment he means Lawrence.

'Peter Pan.'

'No.' I sigh. 'And I never have been.'

'I didn't ever get that sense with Lawrence, you know. The father of your child. But I always had it with *him*.' Oliver moves his gaze to the window, letting out a breath that fogs on the glass. 'Is this because we couldn't conceive?'

'Of course not.'

He turns to look at me properly now. He always seems unrested these days, his eyes shadowed with weariness. He shaves less often, and his face has filled out slightly, from stress, or age, perhaps a little of both. But now, for the briefest of moments, he appears youthful again, his expression newly animated. As if he doesn't want to break up; as if he does have the energy to try.

Rain reverberates against the car roof, so hard it makes the metal vibrate.

'You know,' he says, 'the idea you have in your head of the perfect relationship, the perfect family, the perfect life . . . it doesn't exist. It never did.'

'I never wanted perfection.'

'Then what did you want?'

'What we had, for a long time. Love. A good life together. Happiness.'

He raps his fingertips on the steering wheel and looks out of the window again. 'So, what's first on the list? Skydive? Fancy haircut? Saga singles holiday?'

'No plans yet,' I say quietly, ignoring his contempt.

He frowns. 'Does Emma know?'

I swallow and nod. 'Yes. But she loves you, Oliver. You've been her second dad, for almost her whole life. Nothing will ever change that.'

'Is it worth us going back to the therapist—?' he begins, then breaks off. A moment passes. 'No. It probably isn't.'

I feel a tiny flare of frustration at this. *You were the one who decided therapy was a waste of time. You were the one who didn't want to try.*

Maybe I will say this to him, one day. But not today.

He starts the engine, then slides the gearstick into reverse before pausing. 'You really think you ever gave me a fair shot, Rachel?'

'For seventeen years? Yes, I think so.'

'Ah. You mean you've served your time.'

SECTION V

75.

Josh

December 2026

'It's good to see you, mate,' I say to Giles, gripping his hand.

Wide-eyed, Giles looks at Lola, then back at me. 'Bloody hell. What's with the funeral face? You know I'm not dead yet?'

I smile. 'Sorry.'

He shakes his head. 'Even *Blake* left his flat for long enough to grace me with his presence yesterday. Things really must be serious.'

'You have just had surgery for cancer, darling,' Lola reminds him.

'Yeah, and they got it all, and the consultant says I have every reason to feel positive.' Giles examines the glass he's holding, the contents of which resemble pond water. 'Not that she was accounting for this, I shouldn't think.'

'Complain all you like, but you're drinking it,' Lola says, before squeezing my shoulder and leaving us alone.

Giles leans towards me, hands me the glass. 'Right. Here's where you get to prove what a good friend you are.'

I smile. 'Very funny.'

He does look healthy today, I think. Freshly shaved and plump-cheeked, a splash of wintry sunlight brightening his skin.

I've always thought getting older kind of suited Giles. He wears the extra years well, invariably seems pretty content and fulfilled – not like those shells of humans who weigh out their granola and steam-clean their erogenous zones. Giles just enjoys himself. He gets what life is for. Which is why this has all seemed so unfair.

I notice a hand-drawn card on his side table. It's of a bandaged heart, Rachel's signature a flourish in the bottom corner. It makes me smile and want to well up, all at the same time.

I lift the glass of gunk. 'Am I allowed to ask what's in it?'

'Probably better you don't know. Although, I'd recommend pinching your nose while you swallow. It tastes like it's been siphoned off a swamp.'

'Well, if you think I'm risking Lola's wrath to drink bog, you must be on the *really* good drugs.'

Giles stares at the glass as if he's hoping it might drain of its own accord. 'Maybe you had it right all along, mate.'

'Had what right?'

He shrugs, almost helplessly. 'You'll never have any of this stuff hanging over you.'

I'd swap my life with yours in a second, I think but don't say. 'You have kids, a loving family,' I remind him. 'People who give a shit if you get ill. Who make you smoothies out of kale. Who fall asleep at your bedside in hospital. Who'll do literally anything to make you laugh.'

Giles brightens momentarily. His twin daughters – my tiny Tolstoy enthusiasts, now twenty-eight – are forever sending him funny videos and stupid GIFs to lift his spirits. Some days, he confided, when he was in the thick of it a few months back, they were all that kept him going.

'You wouldn't rather have cancer.'

'No,' I concede, instantly chastened. Because how can you possibly tell a man in his position that a finite existence is something you envy?

'Anyway. Rachel would do all that stuff for you.'

'She might have done, once.'

Giles leans forward, taps his index finger against the table. 'Don't tell Lo, but I've been looking into all that plasma stuff.'

I have a feeling I know what's coming. 'Don't you think that all feels a bit . . . you know. Cannibalistic?'

'If cannibalism is what it takes to get a second lease of life, I'm down with it.'

'You've already got a second lease of life,' I remind him softly.

'You could give me *your* plasma.' The expression on his face straddles that fraying line between humour and hope. 'Kind of like donating a kidney. Only less invasive.'

'Giles—'

'I'd offer you mine in return, but I don't think you'd want it.'

It's funny, really. There was a time when I might have. But I no longer crave to be restored to the age I should be, and definitely not via being jabbed with an older man's bodily fluids.

'Tell you what,' I say, 'if you ever need my spare kidney, it's yours.'

'I tell *you* what. It's nice to have you back.'

'What? I never went anywhere.'

Giles taps the side of his head. 'In here. Thought we'd lost you for a while. It's nice to see you living for you again. If you know what I mean.'

He's only partly right, but I appreciate the sentiment. 'I thought I'd lost me too, for a while, actually. Thanks for kicking me up the arse that time.'

He nods solemnly, then lifts his hand, and we bump fists.

'You ever hear from Wilf?' he asks.

How is it that the softest of syllables can still feel so sharp? It's a long time since Giles has mentioned Wilf's name. But perhaps coming close to death has reanimated all the loose ends of his life to date. So maybe I owe him the truth now, about how it all went down. The real reason Wilf left the country.

But I still feel a kind of animal loyalty towards Wilf, despite our standoff. He sacrificed his own life, really, for mine. And, as far as I know, he remains the only other person on the planet who has been frozen in time. Which means that one day, I hope, he might be open to resurrecting the friendship we once had.

So eventually, I just shake my head and say, 'Not for years.'

Without commenting further, Giles rubs a hand through his greying hair. 'So, come on. When's *Graveyard Heart: The Movie* out? I need something to look forward to.'

I tell him not any time soon, because we've run into problems with financing. But the serialisation of one of my older crime novels is just about to start shooting, and I'm finishing up a new standalone book, my eighth. My newfound readership has been clamouring for more love stories. But, having wrestled pretty hard with writing the sequel to *Graveyard Heart*, on that front right now I'm pretty much spent.

Melvin retired just before Christmas, so I have a new, hotshot-type agent representing me, who's smart and responsive and brokers deals like a demon. I know how lucky I am, professionally speaking. I reflect on it every day. But, at the same time, I have come to realise that superficial success – the type that people often envy – comes nowhere close to family, love, the absolute hands-down privilege of getting old.

The gifts people take for granted – which to them might seem unremarkable – increasingly feel like the most magical things to me.

* * *

I catch Lola in the kitchen on my way out. The worktop is weighed down now by unpalatable-looking cookbooks, giant tubs of pulses, an industrial-sized juicer.

I pull her into a hug. She is tiny and slight in my arms, and her heart is beating fast. She's always complaining about feeling old, but, every time, I tell her I envy her crow's feet and smile lines, the speckles of grey in her hair. All signs, to me, of a life well-lived.

'You didn't drink that juice for him, did you?' she mumbles into my chest.

'The quagmire-in-a-glass? What do you think?'

'Breathe,' she orders, pulling back and putting her face close to mine.

I laugh and oblige.

She tries to laugh too. But then her eyes fill up suddenly, a sharp tide of overwhelm. 'I don't know what I'd do without him, Josh.'

I pull her back into my arms. 'Hey. Hey. You don't have to think like that. He's doing really well. You're going to be okay, I promise.'

We just stand there for a while as I hold her.

'I heard what you were saying. About wishing you had a family.'

'Forget it, Lo,' I murmur.

'Josh, a family can be whatever you want it to be. It's not about blood, or biology. You create your family. A love like that . . . it's made, not inherited. You have our girls, and Polly's boys, and Emma. Don't you see?'

'Better go,' I whisper, blinking back fresh emotion. 'I'm teaching in a bit.'

'I saw Rach yesterday,' she says, as I'm pulling on my coat and scarf. 'She's found a new house.'

'That's good. She okay?'

'You should get in touch.'

My mind journeys back in time nearly twenty-two years. Darren doing his Superman impression. *You get what I'm saying. Just give her some time.*

'I'll wait till she gets in touch with me,' I say to Lola.

A wry smile. 'Still playing that game?'

'I just don't want her to think—'

'She doesn't think anything. But she does need all the friends she can get right now.'

76.

Rachel

June 2027

For our birthday, Josh invites me out to lunch. Nothing fancy, but nice enough to feel like an occasion.

Now that we live less than ten minutes apart, we've been seeing each other a fair bit, for coffee and brunch dates, dinner, movie nights. If Emma's around, she tags along too. I love watching her and Josh spend time together, catching up and making each other laugh, swapping stories about me.

Today, though, it's just the two of us. Which is equally lovely. Time and smiles shared across a table, still my favourite thing to do after nearly forty years of knowing him.

He is telling me about his holiday. He has just come back from a fortnight in the Bahamas, newly suntanned and enviably refreshed. He invited me to go too, when he first booked the tickets. Emma was adamant I should accept, even threatening to say yes on my behalf. But in the end there were too many reasons not to. The romance of the resort. The idea of people staring at us, lying on a beach together. The myriad complications of swimsuits and alcohol and two weeks alone with Josh while still, in my heart, knowing him to be the most handsome man in any room. Or poolside cabana, come to that.

He asks after Emma now, and I tell him she's waiting to find out if she will gain tenancy with the Gray's Inn chambers where she's been working as a pupil barrister. The pressure to perform has been fierce; I don't think she's slept more than three hours a night for almost a full year. But soon my baby, who was once no bigger than a blueberry, could be defending criminals in a court of law for a living.

The waiter brings over our drinks and a basket of warm rolls. I take one and smother whipped butter on to it, though I have to break it into pieces, because my dentist has ordered me to stop tearing bread apart with my teeth.

'Do you think you could ever put weight on?' I ask Josh.

'Er, I don't think so. Not in the same way as other people. Why?'

'I don't know. I was thinking about how you always wear the same pair of jeans.'

Yes – always the same jeans and slate-grey T-shirt, dark hair persistently shambolic. Endearingly uncomplicated, doing his best to blend in.

'You mean, the same *kind* of jeans. I have more than one pair, Rach.'

'Well, it must be nice, anyway. Not to have to worry about it.'

'Yeah, I'll add it to my list of minor upsides.' A pause. 'Hey, you know my crime series airs in a couple of months?'

'Of course. It's on the calendar in glitter pen,' I say with a smile.

'There's a premiere in London. Will you come?'

The smile fades a little. 'Ah, I couldn't.'

'What? Why not?'

'Because, Josh.'

'Because what?'

'*Because*, everyone will assume I'm your mother.'

We both reach for the water jug, and, as we do, it's hard not to notice the disparity between his seamless, silicone skin and mine. On me, the passing years are unmissable, my lines and emerging liver spots like tiny time stamps. A reminder, if we needed one, of the chasm between us now that can never be crossed.

Josh doesn't press me further. So perhaps he is seeing it too.

I'm not self-conscious, particularly. But I am aware of my changing body, in a detached, almost fascinated, way, I suppose. Stretch marks, tits losing their bounce, glimmers of silver visible in my hair if I stand beneath bright light. My limbs starting to thicken too, perhaps, ever so slightly.

Not long ago, Josh told me he finally came clean about his true age with his new agent and publisher. Fortunately, the huge bestseller he wrote means he had the leverage to swear them all to secrecy.

'Do you ever worry about the future?' I ask him.

'Sure. But at some point it'll become meaningless, right?'

'That's a bit nihilistic.'

'Well, once you're gone, and Emma's . . . There'll come a time when . . .'

In my heart, a faultline begins to form. 'There'll come a time when what?'

He hesitates. 'Let's not talk about all that stuff. It's our birthday. We're supposed to be having fun.'

Shortly after this, I go to the toilet, where I bump into a woman who's clearly steaming drunk. Her eyes are glazed, and her cheeks are raspberry-red. She's about my age, possibly slightly older.

'Tell me your secret,' she says, laying a heavy hand on my arm.

I smile uncertainly. 'Sorry?'

'My lad won't be seen dead with me. I'm lucky if I even get a birthday card from him these days.'

Her assumption rocks me. 'Oh, that's not—'

'No – you should give yourself credit.' The smile drops from her face slightly. 'You must have been a really good mum.'

And then she leaves, bouncing off the door frame as she sways her way back to her table.

Josh walks me home, and I invite him in for coffee. Once we're sitting on the sofa, I relate the story to him about the loo woman, at which he starts laughing.

I pick up a cushion, sling it gently into his ribs. 'It's exactly why I can't go to that premiere with you. She thought you were my *son*. I can't believe you don't find that disturbing.'

The smile leaves his face in a way that looks like self-reproach. 'Well, of course I do. Of course we couldn't have lived with that. You're right, Rach. You always are.'

I rest my head on his shoulder, the worn-in cotton of his T-shirt. I feel his heartbeat against my cheek, a soft strike in time with mine.

'You know,' he murmurs, his chin grazing my hair, 'every morning, when I wake up, I hope – just for a second – that I dreamed this whole thing. That I'm going to see your face smiling on the pillow next to me, eighteen all over again.'

The late-afternoon light has dipped. The room is dimmer and soundless now, but in a way that feels comforting and safe. A place with no clocks, bright lights, or expectations. Where the world can be withheld, if only for a few hours.

Josh puts his arms around me, tugs me close. 'In another life, Rach,' he whispers.

My heart feels whole and broken all at once. 'In another life,' I whisper back.

77.

Josh

June 2028

I've been debating going into hiding ever since Emma – for reasons best known to herself – began talking about throwing Rachel and me 'a big fuck-off party' for our fifty-eighth birthday. Quite why she's decided now is the time to jump-start our social lives I have no idea, but Rachel thinks it was after she mentioned to Emma that she'd been thinking of joining the National Trust.

Fortunately, Polly ends up thwarting Emma's sociopathic intentions by inviting the three of us to her middle son Fred's wedding, that same weekend.

On top of my general aversion to birthdays, I'm not normally a fan of large social gatherings where more than a few people know me. Someone usually feels the need to single me out and remark upon how young I look, or tell me how much they hated the ending to one – or all – of my books or TV shows.

But, given there will be cake, champagne and – if all goes to plan – a party atmosphere, I decide to accept the invite. Mostly in order to get Emma off my back.

It's surreal sometimes, spending time with Rachel's daughter. She probably doesn't remember that, growing up, she used to be my little buddy. I could lift her up with one hand, make her squeal with laughter just by pulling a stupid face. I have read to her, done jigsaws with her, let her eat Nutella from the jar with her fist. Taken her swimming, pushed her on countless swings.

Now, though, biologically, we are only five years apart.

The dinner and speeches are over, which is a relief for all one hundred and fifty of us, because Fred's best man – who's old enough to know better – seemed only to be familiar with jokes that stopped being funny in the eighties.

In front of us they're setting up a dance floor, which I fully plan to ignore, because there's one thing that pill never fixed, and that's being afflicted with worse co-ordination than your average newborn foal.

'Well, here's to you both,' Emma says, raising her glass. We are drinking champagne, Emma having insisted on buying a bottle from the marquee bar. 'How does it feel to be fifty-eight?'

Rachel sips her drink and smiles. 'Better if you stop saying fifty-eight.'

'Am I going to see the pair of you up on that dance floor later?'

'Nobody wants to see that,' Rachel and I say, at exactly the same time.

We chat for a while longer, then Rachel says, with an oddly conspiratorial smile, 'Hey, do you reckon anyone here thinks you're my daughter and son?'

'Jesus, can we not,' I say urgently.

'Or maybe they think we're boyfriend and girlfriend,' Emma says, throwing me an exaggerated wink.

I pretend to check my phone. 'They said carriages at three, yes?'

Rachel laughs and squeezes my arm. 'Sorry, sorry.' She turns to her daughter. 'How about you tell us about your actual boyfriend?'

'Mum, we've been through this. George isn't my boyfriend.'

'Oh, sorry. Of course. What would you call him, then?'

'An acquaintance. As in, a solicitor I quite like and occasionally sleep with.'

Rachel makes a pleading face. 'Can I meet him?'

'Absolutely, if you're arrested for a crime. Be sure to call Morton and Whittaker and ask for George Holdsworth.'

Rachel sighs, defeated.

Predictably, Emma turns to me. 'How about you, Josh? Anyone you're occasionally sleeping with?'

'Nope. Too tired for all that now.'

'Tired?'

'Up here.' I tap the side of my head.

'I thought your brain hadn't aged a day in nearly three decades.'

'No. But I've lived every one of them. It's mental, not physical.'

'Isn't that why you do yoga and wash exclusively in cold water?'

I smile, tempted to remind her there are some types of tiredness that exercise and ice baths can't touch. But that's the kind of defeatist talk she likes to tell me off for.

'If Josh is tired, then I should definitely be feeling my age,' Rachel says.

'*Should*, bollocks.' Emma tips back some champagne. 'You feel how you feel. And you feel great, don't you?'

Rachel shrugs. 'Yes, mostly.'

'Good,' Emma says. 'Then let's talk holidays. It's looking as if I might have a window towards the end of the year.'

A few months ago, Emma officially mooted the idea of the three of us going away together. Rachel has turned down the last couple of trips I've proposed, but, once I extended the invitation to Emma too, she seemed more open to the prospect. In the end, though, Emma's work calendar transpired to be blocked out for the foreseeable future. Since securing tenancy last year she hasn't had a break that's lasted longer than five minutes, as far as I can work out. I asked her once when she'll be allowed to take her foot off the pedal, whereupon she shot me a withering look and said, 'When I retire.'

'Where do you fancy?' says Rachel.

Emma turns to me. 'Any ideas, globetrotter?'

As nicknames go, it could be worse. I have been travelling a fair bit lately, ever since I caved and paid someone dodgy for a passport with a birth date that finally tallied with my face. 'Wherever you like. I'm easy. You decide.'

'Hmm. I don't know. Maybe somewhere like ... Aruba?' Emma says.

She got it out of me, once. That Aruba was a place I'd wanted to go with Rachel.

I shoot her a *stop it* look. But she just beams at me.

Thankfully, Rachel appears not to notice, and the moment moves on.

I sit at the edge of the dance floor until well into the evening. Rachel and Emma come and go, mingling and catching up. Fortunately, aside from the odd exchange of pleasantries, I'm largely left alone. Maybe people don't make the connection with the fifty-something geezer I should be when they see me. Or maybe they do, and have no idea what to say.

The band switches tempo to something slow. A step back in time, to nineties-era Westlife. A blast from a golden past.

As the music kicks in, Rachel appears in front of me, her hand outstretched. There are nearly thirty years between us tonight, but I think – not for the first time – that she looks beautiful as ever. She's teased a curl through her hair, which is short now but still blonde, albeit slowly greying along the crown. Her dress is a medley of fuchsia and peach, pleated from the waist, and her lips are a riotous pink. She is, as she always has been, dazzling.

Still. No need to kill the moment with a dance. I smile at her, shake my head. 'Ah, no. We scare people on dance floors, remember?'

'Don't worry.' She returns my smile. 'They're bound to look at the two of us and blame me.'

And so, as sunset submits to dusk, and the canopy of lights flares gold, I follow Rachel on to the dance floor. The outdoor air is perfumed with dampening grass, slumbering rose bushes.

I pull her close, wrap my arms around her back. The kite-high pleasure of being close to her like this is something I'd filed into the deepest recesses of my memory. I'm not really ready for what it does to me. She lays her head on my shoulder, and I feel loss blow through me, sharp as a winter wind.

'Love you,' I whisper, into the soft folds of her hair.

'Love you too,' she whispers back.

As the music plays on and we slowly turn around together, I catch sight of Emma watching us, her phone lifted to capture the moment.

She brushes something from her cheek, and I shut my eyes.

78.

Rachel

June 2030

To celebrate my turning sixty, Emma books dinner for the two of us at her favourite restaurant in London.

I catch the train in, having agreed to meet Emma at her flat. But when I emerge from the tube station – as I have done a thousand times before – it is as though my mind has violently upturned with a mental bout of vertigo.

It seems, all at once, an impossible feat to get to the flat from where I am. There are too many things required of me – navigating a crowd, remembering the way. I feel, strongly, as if I need to hold on to someone, or something. My clothes feel horribly tight, appearing to have shrunk around my body since only this morning. I stand and tug at my collar, to try to free up some air.

A stranger pushes past me, knocking my shoulder. He tuts, and I startle, my breath picking up pace. I am reminded, suddenly, of that sticker they put on hire car wing mirrors. *Objects are closer than they appear.*

The air is hot, seeming fast and thunderously loud, as if I have found myself standing next to a runway.

I plant my feet, trying to steady myself and think. Do I turn left or right to get to Emma's flat? The information is there – I can *feel* it, like an object rolled beneath a piece of furniture, but I cannot make my mind stretch quite far enough to reach it.

Still Falling For You

I have a map on my phone, but it seems incredible that I should need to use it. And anyway, the prospect of doing so only adds to the jumble in my mind.

The world appears to shrink, pavements and concrete and clouds closing in.

My phone rings, and I answer it with a jolt.

'Mum, how are you getting on?' Emma has booked dinner at seven o'clock in town, and I am already late because the train was delayed.

'Is it left, or right?' My voice seems to be doing its own thing, the words emerging awkwardly in lumps.

There is a short pause. 'Is what left or right?'

'From the station,' I say impatiently. 'Do I turn left, or right?'

'Right,' she says slowly. 'Then first left. Like always.'

I turn to look at the sign behind me. I can feel my confidence – hard-won, over the years – beginning to fade. It is frustrating as a phone signal that has weakened without warning. Is this how it feels to turn sixty?

'And it is Kilburn, isn't it?'

A pause. 'Sorry?'

'Is Kilburn the right station?'

'You know what, Mum? Stay there. Don't move. I'm coming to get you.'

Over dinner at the sushi place Emma loves in St Paul's, she tells me Oliver has a new girlfriend.

Though our parting wasn't easy, he and I still speak from time to time, on birthdays and at Christmas, other special occasions. And I am relieved and happy that he has remained very close to Emma.

After she's filled me in, Emma says, 'Mum . . . what was all that about earlier? At the station.'

By the time she reached me I'd become quite distressed. So much so that, when I saw her, I burst into sobs so forceful they shocked us both.

'I'm sorry, sweetheart. I didn't mean to upset you. It's just an ageing thing, I think.' Because, I have had to conclude on a few occasions over the past couple of years, that's what it must be.

'You're sixty. Not to mention the least flappable person I've ever met.'

'Still. It happens, from time to time.'

'Does it?' She picks up her wine glass. 'Like, what kind of thing?'

I prepare to dither while I think of a good example, but am surprised to find one comes easily. 'Well, the other day, I was waiting at a junction and I couldn't remember what side of the road to drive on. I just . . . couldn't remember.'

'Mum.' Emma leans forward, eyes abruptly wide. 'Are you serious?'

'Oh, it only lasted a few seconds. Until I saw some other cars, then I was fine.'

'Until you saw some other cars then you were fine?' she repeats, leaning on the words in a way that's oddly reminiscent of her father being obtuse.

'I'm making it sound worse than it was. Just a momentary lapse.' I put my hand over hers. 'You worry too much. I had it when I was pregnant with you as well. Baby brain, they used to call it.'

'But . . . you're not pregnant now.'

I sip my wine. *What a strange comment*, I think.

'No,' I say eventually, to humour her more than anything else. 'You're right. I'm not.'

* * *

Later, for the first time, we go through my pregnancy sketchbook together. I brought it with me this weekend to show her, although I almost left it behind on the train.

Lawrence's hand on my stomach, a few months in. The first sleepsuit we chose together. The cucumbers I kept insisting on eating whole. Her teddy bear, the one she still has on a shelf above her bed. Lawrence building her cot. My expanding belly. The night-time view from her little nursery window.

At one of the pages, Emma pauses. 'This has been ripped out.'

I swallow, remembering the realisation that I had sketched Josh with his feet up reading a baby book, instead of her father.

She holds my gaze with a faint smile, eyes lunar-pale in the half-light. 'It's funny. You'd never know from these that Dad was totally the wrong person for you.'

'Emma,' I say – and I will keep repeating myself on this, no matter how many times she needs to hear it – 'if I hadn't been with him, then I never would have had you. So I don't have a single regret about how things worked out. Not one.'

79.

Josh

August 2030

Rachel and I go out for lunch at the kind of pub we used to love when we were married. It has a huge beer garden that rambles down to the river, serves platefuls of food so big they leave you semi-comatose.

The lawn is almost full, with only a table beneath a lime tree going free. Everyone else is basking in the sun, limbs bare and faces upturned, as we might have once too, forty-odd years ago. Nowadays, I'm much more like a dog, seeking out shade whenever I can.

Rachel took some persuading, to come here today. She's been telling me a lot lately that she prefers to do things at her own pace. Which is odd, because my life is hardly a non-stop bender. She's turned down a couple of parties recently, and has become increasingly impatient with Ingrid, who keeps trying to get her to fly out to LA. Rachel insists she's tired, that she's taken on too much work over the past few months, and has struggled to get over a particularly nasty bout of flu.

She has just said – again – that she thinks she looks old enough to be my mother. Even though she knows I hate it when she talks like this.

'Well, you don't. But even if you did, who cares?'

The correct answer to this is no one. I don't, and I can't believe Rachel still gives a shit. And there is not a person in this beer garden who has slung more than a brief glance our way since we got here.

'I'm going to ask someone.'

'Rach—'

'Excuse me,' Rachel says sweetly to a passing server, while I consider if there is time to secrete myself beneath the table before he sees me. 'Can I ask you something?'

The kid is young, maybe twenty. Then again, these days it's becoming harder and harder to tell. Kids are getting Botox in their teens.

I pull my sunglasses firmly down over my face.

'Yes?' the server says uncertainly, looking between the two of us.

'Me and this man,' Rachel says, gesturing in my direction. 'What would you say our relationship is?'

'I don't know,' the boy says nervously, shading his eyes against the sun. 'Nan?'

Despite myself, I suppress a laugh.

'Thank you,' Rachel says to him. 'You've been most helpful.'

The kid walks away, and Rachel turns back to face me. 'Nan,' she deadpans.

I notice, suddenly, that her shirt is misbuttoned. But I decide against telling her. It's not gaping or anything. Just a mistake. Unusually, I sense – for some reason – that my pointing it out might embarrass her.

'Well, cheers for establishing that,' I say. 'Though I don't know why you felt the need to drag an innocent child into it.'

'Oh, he loved it.' She throws me an exaggerated wink.

Something's off.

The thought hits without warning, alarming as a brick through glass.

I've not seen Rachel for a couple of months. But, today, she is different. I sense it now, not with my mind, but with my body. The knock of my pulse, the hairs going hard on my arms.

Rachel has never been the type of person to ask strangers to referee debates between us. Or amuse herself, but no one else, with *Carry On* winks. She used to groan at innuendo, and not in an appreciative way.

And there is something else. Something about the expression on her face. The way her eyes don't quite land on me. As though we're at opposite ends of a telescope, our proximity just illusion.

She raps her fingers on the table, looks distractedly away from me across the garden.

'Hey,' Emma says briskly.

'Hey. You got five minutes?'

'Not really. Two, maybe. Insane deadlines. You know how it is.'

I do. But I suspect hers are slightly more pressing than mine, given that they involve things like court dates and murderers.

'What's up?' she says.

I picture Emma tight-jawed at her laptop, head in the law and not at all where I am. 'I met your mum for lunch today.'

'Oh, yeah. Nice time?'

'Yeah, thanks. But I wanted to ask . . . does she seem different to you, at all?'

I hear fear in the pause that follows. 'What do you mean?' But I know she knows, because she says this so quietly, the words emerge barely formed.

My eyes stray to the first-edition copy of *The Remains of the Day* Rachel gave me for Christmas, two whole decades ago now. I reach up and take it down from the shelf, then thumb gently through it, as I do sometimes when I'm thinking of her.

I realise I cannot find the language to describe the shape and colour of the foreboding inside me. Slippery as shadow, dark as nightfall.

'I think something's wrong.'

On the end of the line, Emma lets out a long breath. And there it is: my worst fears confirmed. 'I think something's wrong too. She's not herself.'

'No. There are moments when—'

'Oh, my God, Josh.' Emma's voice sounds suddenly muffled, as if she has covered her mouth as the shock finally surfaces.

I shut the book, stare down at the image of the pocket watch on the cover. It overwhelms me suddenly, the inevitability of time passing.

'No, this can't be . . . She's too young,' Emma says.

I think of Rachel's mother. 'She isn't,' I whisper.

'Fuck.' Her voice is pitched high, tiny and terrified.

'It'll be okay.'

'How can you know that?'

'Because. It has to be,' is all I say.

80.

Rachel

September 2030

The moment I know – I mean, *really* know – comes on an innocuous Tuesday in September.

It started almost as imperceptibly as the drip from a tap – so soft and sporadic, I neglected to pay attention at first. It just didn't seem like something that needed fixing. Words and places falling, very occasionally, out of my head. Emails unintentionally not responded to. Insurances lapsing. Getting lost on the way into town. Struggling to plant my feet on the stairs. Failing for a minute or so to place my godchild – Lo's daughter – when she messaged me last month. Forgetting Ingrid's birthday, which I have never done before in my life. And then trying to blame it on the time difference, which – as Polly gently pointed out – made absolutely no sense at all.

And now, after searching for nearly a full morning, I open the bathroom cabinet to find my wallet on the second shelf.

I stare at it in shock, like I have stumbled upon a wasp's nest. *When, and why?* I have no recollection at all of putting it in here.

I feel my cheeks flush red. Because, even though I am alone and unobserved, the humiliation roars.

I have recently turned sixty, which is hardly old, of course. But I feel there is a ghoulishness to the world's preoccupation with the ageing body. There are certainly enough adverts and doctors and newspaper headlines and segments on daytime

Still Falling For You

television that seem, to me, absurdly sensationalist. I find the narrative petty and dull, so I generally ignore it. Life has been kind to me, and I am lucky. And, as my friends and I so often say, it makes absolutely no sense that we should pay attention to the people who try to sell us fear.

Ingrid has mentioned a couple of times lately that she thinks I've lost my spark. She's asked if it's because I don't like getting older. But ageing doesn't trouble me – it is normal and expected that I should experience the occasional twinge in my back, and that it takes me longer than it once did to recover from a jog. Admittedly I am more precautionary, these days: I've cut down on alcohol, and have started lifting light weights, on the advice of Josh, ever since Lo slipped a disc shaving her legs. I never did get the hang of yoga, much as I tried.

But I do not resent these things. To do so would be like begrudging sunrise, or the turn of the seasons, the twist of a tide.

That said, I have been keeping a kind of diary recently. On the first page, I headed it *Things of Mild Concern*. And much of what I have recorded so far, I've begun to realise, has been a series of little memory lapses – circuit-breaks and gaps in my thinking, like bricks missing in a building. My mind sometimes resembles one of those computer games where the floor opens up without warning, cleaving maliciously apart. And I need to concentrate, hard, so I don't fall into the darkness that is waiting.

After retrieving my wallet, I make a coffee and take a biscuit from the tin, and then another. I force myself to go through the rigmarole of my weekly online shop, then exchange some messages with Emma, and one with Lawrence. He's back in Bedford next week on a flying visit from the Cotswolds, where he lives now with his girlfriend. He is keen for us all to go out for dinner, but I decide I don't want to see him. I couldn't bear it if something embarrassing were to happen in front of him.

By the time I can bring myself to jot down the wallet incident in my notebook, it is almost dark.

Once I'm finished, I get out my phone. I know Josh is busy right now, writing his next book, and with a TV series in pre-production. But I would like, I think, to feel reassured by him.

Or perhaps it is not reassurance I want. Perhaps, in fact, it is honesty.

I have been telling myself – over and over – that I am too young for this to be happening. If my mother ever enters my mind, I push her swiftly away, as I have been used to doing for much of the past fifty years.

But ignoring the truth is never more than a temporary fix. Reality is guaranteed to return, the way a dead body will always rise to the surface of a lake.

I scroll down to Josh's name, double-checking I've remembered it right, since I seem to be in the habit of misdialling people lately.

But, as my fingers hover over his name, I feel a chill of fear seep slowly through me, pooling in voids I didn't know existed.

In my hand, I let the screen fade to black.

81.

Rachel

August 2031

Thirteen years after *Graveyard Heart* was first published, the film is finally released.

Josh invites me to the premiere in London. For weeks he tag-teams with Emma on trying to persuade me. But I am resolute. I know there's no way I could walk a red carpet with him now, no matter how meaningful the occasion. I have to do things at my own pace these days, in private, well away from the glare of observation. I haven't told him I've been struggling for balance recently, reluctant to leave the house in case I topple and hit my head. The thought of doing so at an event in front of cameras is almost unbearable. Most of the time, I'm worried people might assume I'm drunk.

In the end, we agree to go together to see it at the cinema.

I am late, of course, as I so often am now. I end up doing two laps of the block before I see that Josh has come outside the cinema to wait for me and I remember what it is I am meant to be doing. But I brazen it out – just apologise, and pretend the bus was delayed.

Before the film starts, as the cinema plays a needlessly explosive advert for a new streaming service, I lean over and say to Josh, 'I need to ask you something. It's to do with Emma.'

'Sure,' he says, through a mouthful of popcorn. He extends the carton to me, but I shake my head. The last time I ate popcorn, I cracked a tooth on a rogue kernel and had to pay an extortionate amount of money for emergency dental work.

'I need you to promise that . . . if anything happens to me, you'll look after her. Properly take care of her. Whatever she needs.'

I see him swallow, a muscle leap in his neck. 'I really hate it when you say shit like that, Rach.'

'She would need you, though. If I wasn't here.'

'Ah, she wouldn't. Fussing around her like some tragic long-lost uncle.'

It's funny, because I think Josh often *feels* like a sixty-something now, just as I do. Not in his body, but his soul.

'You know I'd be there for her,' he says. 'That's a given. But Emma . . . she's strong.'

I feel myself starting to get worked up. It can happen so quickly these days. 'She isn't always,' I insist. 'And especially after Lawrence . . .'

Lawrence had a heart attack last year, but – true to form – he responded as though it had been nothing more than a mild inconvenience, like sunburn, or a hangover. He broke up with his long-term girlfriend shortly afterwards, and has apparently been partying hard ever since. And I know it worries Emma.

The trailers draw to a close, and all the lights go out.

Josh reaches for my hand in the blackness, wrapping his fingers over mine. The way he used to in cinemas, back when we were married. I would feel for the writer's bump on his finger, eating white-chocolate jazzies with my free hand, and my heart in the dark would be bright as a summer sky.

'Look,' Josh whispers, 'this hardly needs to be said. But you know I would take care of Emma.'

'Promise?'

'I promise.'

The music starts, and the opening credits come up. *Based on the bestselling novel by Josh Foster.*

'Hey,' I whisper, my heart swelling with pride. 'It's you.'

The film begins, but he doesn't let go of my hand.

It's late when we get out, so Josh drops me back at home, where we come to a pause together in the hallway.

His eyes are filled with tears, and he asks me the question without words.

I just nod.

A few months back, following gentle but persistent pressure from Emma and Josh and my friends, I went with Emma to see one of Lo's daughters, now a GP. I probably downplayed my difficulties, in the hope that she might say I had nothing to worry about. But she seemed concerned enough to refer me. And now, after a series of scans and appointments with three different specialists, it has been confirmed. The changes in my brain have been made official. They can no longer be argued with.

Josh drops to the floor in a crouch, puts his head in his hands.

With some effort, I lower myself to join him, slipping my arms around his back. He inclines right into me, grips me tight. And then we just sit there for a while, our bodies a warm knot on the cold hallway tiles. It takes me right back to that morning we hid in a wardrobe together, on New Year's Day a million years ago.

It is agonising, the idea that these memories will one day start to fade. I want to cling to them – little lifebelts that might save me from disappearing completely – for as long as I can.

Eventually, I laugh softly. 'Maybe I should have taken that second pill after all. I went to my own mother's funeral, but I still never thought it could happen to me.' I shake my head. 'I was *determined* it wouldn't happen to me.'

And of course I know it's not a question of willpower. But I still feel determined, just in a different way. I am determined not to fear this. Because I have seen, long ago, what fear can do to a person.

In my arms, Josh turns to look at me.

'Don't say it.'

He smiles, the softest of smiles. And then he blinks, a single tear slipping free. 'Wouldn't dream of it.'

After that, we remain where we are on the floor together, talking until the light has long-since sunk from the sky. He makes tiny, tender confessions. Things I never knew before. I do the same. And, as we trade feelings and memories, the world – for the first time in a while – begins to feel normal again. Less warped, no longer a labyrinth.

Just how it always was.

Eventually, because I really do get quite tired these days, I find myself drifting towards sleep. Josh is telling me about his flat, something to do with those paint samples on his bedroom wall still being in situ, nearly three decades on. 'Turns out it's too hard to decide between vanilla and vanilla,' he says, and I smile, and the last thing I hear as I close my eyes is the sound of his voice.

It is, I think, the last sound I would ever want to hear.

82.

Rachel

July 2033

I seem to have got into the habit of upsetting people lately, one way or another. And today is no different.

Josh is here, and he has brought a picnic. After we've eaten, we lie on a rug in my back garden, side by side beneath an old parasol I'd forgotten I had. The day feels companionable and safe, the sky endlessly blue.

Suddenly, I sit up. There is something buzzing nearby, a grinding, repetitive whirring. An insect? But I can't see it. I wonder how big it might be, to be capable of making a noise so jarring.

'You okay?' Josh says, sitting up too.

'What's that noise?'

It takes him a long time to answer, so maybe he is also confused. 'A lawnmower,' he says eventually. 'Someone's mowing their lawn.'

'Who is?'

'One of your neighbours?'

He says this as if he's asking me, but I asked him first, so that doesn't make sense. After a moment or two, I give up and just shrug.

The sun is starting to sneak past the edge of the parasol. It feels good against my skin, like something my body needs. Perhaps it will burn off all the fogginess that seems to sit in clumps around my brain these days.

I splay my hand on the grass, press down against the ground. It is hotter than I expected, because it looks so cold and fresh. The lawn and trees and sky are all deep green or vibrant blue. But those colours feel like a lie.

I lift my sunglasses and peer at Josh. It occurs to me that he looks very young, in that tight T-shirt, with his thick, dark hair and boyish, gleaming skin. 'How old are you?'

'Um.' He clears his throat. 'Why do you ask?'

'You look young. How long have we been friends?'

I am surprised to realise he seems emotional suddenly. Tears have bunched in his eyes, and I see him gently clench a fist. Was it something I said?

I suppose it must have been.

He leans over, tugging me into a soft hug. I don't mind: he asks permission with his arms. And he smells very nice, of a fragrance so familiar it feels like time travel.

I smile. Yes, of course. How could I have forgotten? We were married, once.

'A long time,' he murmurs, before pulling back and looking at me with shining eyes. They begin to brim over now, tears turning to raindrops on his face. 'A really long time. Oh, I love you. I love you so much.'

'Why are you crying?' I say, reaching up and dabbing at his cheek with my finger. If I've said something to upset him, I really didn't mean to.

83.

Josh

November 2034

Sitting with Rachel at her house, I pick up a magazine. It's one of those quaint titles about living well, filled with wholesome articles on baking and wild swimming and foraging for things to put in soups. I read to her about a woman who hand-illustrates cookbooks, in the hope that it might spark a sleeping synapse in her brain, deliver her some subconscious pleasure.

She can still read, if the mood takes her. But it so rarely does, these days. I know she's starting to find language confusing, partly because the way she spells is becoming increasingly phonetic.

Before very long, she falls asleep. I just sit next to her and watch her breathing for a while. Then, softly, I take her hand. It feels featherweight and fragile, bird-like, in my own. And I shut my eyes too.

When I stir, Emma is in the armchair opposite us.

'Took a picture,' she says with a smile, lifting her phone. 'Hope you don't mind. The two of you looked so sweet there together.'

Rachel is still dozing, head tipped to one side. I shuffle upright, gently unclasp her hand. She is beautiful as ever, her pale skin sliced with winter sunlight. The room is warm and smells homely, of cooked food and chopped wood ready for the fire.

'I've been trying to do a bit of forward-planning,' Emma says.

Like mother, like daughter, I guess.

'She's deteriorating quite fast.'

I swallow and nod, albeit I try – even now – not to believe it. To hang on to the hope that Rachel will somehow stabilise. Or that we're only imagining how swiftly she's changing. Or that the miracle cure the media outlets keep taunting us with has finally moved beyond trial stage.

In desperation, I even sent an email to Wilf last week, begging him to bring his massive brain out of retirement and invent a way to save her. But my message bounced straight back.

'I was thinking about having Mum come to live with me in London,' Emma says. 'But everyone seems to think it's better for her to be in familiar surroundings, with her garden, and people around who understand the situation, you know? London would be too overwhelming, I think. And the doctor said it might actually cause her to decline more rapidly.'

'I'll do it,' I say, the words almost outpacing my brain.

She hesitates. 'You'll do what?'

I wonder for a moment if I've overstepped the mark. Then I take in the fearful face of the criminal barrister in front of me and decide I don't care. 'Emma, you should know ... a few years ago, your mum asked me to look after you. If anything happened to her. So, if me helping out would mean you could stay in London, and work, and retain some semblance of normality to your life, I'm more than happy to do it.' Emma spends much of her time on trains or in taxis, wheeling a suitcase between various Crown Courts. And she's less than a decade into her career. Having to worry about caring for Rachel as well must threaten to overwhelm her sometimes. 'I'm pretty sure this is exactly what your mum was talking about, when she asked me to look after you.'

'Why do you say that?' In the winter light, Emma's eyes are iceberg-blue.

'Because . . . I think she knew. For a long time, before we did.'

She swallows hard, nods. 'She kept a notebook.'

Briefly, I avert my gaze, because Emma usually prefers to get emotional without an audience. I glance out of the window towards the wintry garden, kissed now by frost.

Emma sighs. 'The thing is, part of the reason Mum left you is because she wouldn't have been comfortable with this exact scenario. Looking after her involves personal care. I'm sorry, but it wouldn't be right.'

'So, we'll get carers to do that. But let me help in other ways. I'll clean, do the shopping, take her to appointments. I'll sit with her. Whatever you need.'

Emma's eyes get wide. Icebergs turning to oceans. 'Why would you disrupt your entire life to do that? You're busy too.'

She's not wrong. My life has felt more hectic over the past few years than perhaps it ever has. Film promo stuff, my twelfth novel out soon, and the mentoring programme I've recently set up for aspiring writers.

But I'd give it all up in a heartbeat, if Emma asked me to.

'Because I love her,' I say.

84.

Rachel

September 2035

A man is sitting with me, reading from a book. It might be about love, or maybe time, because it has a clock on the cover. But it's hard to be sure, since I can't really follow the storyline. There are too many characters, and I'm struggling to keep track of who's saying what.

I prefer watching TV to reading now. There is a good channel I like, which has soothing films of parks and nature and stories about the nineties. It's so much easier to understand.

The man keeps mentioning someone called Stevens, and someone else called Miss Kenton, and I can't remember for the life of me who these people are. I glance around the living room, in case they are both here and I've forgotten, again.

As I turn in my chair, I feel the man looking at me.

'Are you my grandson?' I ask. He does have that air about him, with his scruffy jeans and ruffled hairdo, and the T-shirt that says Teenage Fanclub, which sort of gives him away.

He shakes his head. 'We actually . . . used to be married, a long time ago.'

What a ridiculous thing to say. 'You're far too young for me.'

'Well, yes. I am now, I suppose.'

I have no idea what he's talking about.

It begins to rise again now. The worry that has been nagging at me for a while. 'Have you seen my rings?' I raise my left hand, agitation churning inside me. 'I had two rings, and they're missing. Someone must have taken them.'

As he starts to speak, my eyes stray to his wrist. He is wearing a watch, something silvery in steel. It looks familiar, somehow. I'm sure I saw it in a shop once, agonised over buying it.

'I bought that,' I say slowly, the memory returning to me in darts and flashes.

'You did,' he replies, following my gaze. 'For my birthday, the year I turned thirty.'

I smile, feeling something warm beating in my belly. Happiness, I realise, because I so rarely get things right, these days.

Emma's here now, but she doesn't say hello. She is picking things off the coffee table, dirty cups and newspapers. I don't know who they belong to. Not me: I can't read the paper any more, because the words no longer make sense.

My sketchbook is open on my knee. I look down, but can't make out what it is I've been trying to draw. A dog, maybe. But whose dog? There isn't one here. So maybe it's a watering can.

'Have you seen my rings?'

Emma smiles, seeming not remotely concerned. 'No, but we'll look for them, okay? Why don't you relax for a bit, while lunch is cooking?'

I used to cook quite a lot, but I'm not allowed to use the stove any more, ever since there was some sort of fire last year. There is now a big plastic sign that sits above it: DO NOT USE.

A man puts his head around the door, making me jump.

'Are you here about the fire?' I say, alarmed.

'Mum, it's Josh,' Emma says. 'There's no fire.'

There is a memory fluttering at the back of my mind, to do with this man, but I can't quite pin it down.

Then it comes to me. 'Aruba.' I'm sure he said we were going to Aruba: I have written it in my notebook.

His smile is gentle. People smile at me a lot nowadays, usually as a precursor to correcting me on something, or ordering me about. But I can tell this man's smile is the kind I don't have to worry about.

Suddenly, his face begins to blur with someone else's. Emma's father, perhaps? No, that can't be right. This man is far too young. I really need to start writing these things down. Have I a notebook somewhere?

I tilt my head to get a better look at him, and a bulb in my brain flickers briefly to life, but then quickly blows again.

'Aruba,' he says. 'Yes. We talked about going, once.' But his voice scratches slightly, as though it's hurting him to speak.

Maybe I'll get some fresh air.

I stand up, then hesitate. I can't quite remember the way to the garden. There are far too many rooms in this house. It reminds me of the hospital. I'm always getting lost.

'Everything okay, Mum?'

Sometimes, Emma tells me to draw what I need. But that is ridiculous, obviously, because I'm not a child.

'My rings,' I say, lifting my left hand so she can see. 'Someone's stolen my rings.'

'Ah,' she says mildly, apparently not at all alarmed. Then, 'Would you like some lunch?'

'Yes,' I say, tugging at my collar. It's so stuffy in here. 'I can't remember when I last ate.'

'Please,' the man says.

Please what? I think.

* * *

Still Falling For You

Emma tells me lunch is ready, so I allow her to take me by the arm and help me up. But I feel exhausted: I can barely put one foot in front of the other. I'd really like a lie-down, or maybe to eat lunch from a tray on my lap. Is that really too much to ask?

Suddenly I feel the familiar sensation of beginning to topple. Emma gasps, and I hear a man's voice saying, 'Oh, easy, easy—' and then there are hands beneath my armpits, and everything goes dark.

The next thing I know, I feel as though I'm underwater. I can hear people saying my name but I can't open my eyes. I've wanted to shut them for a long time, I think. It actually feels quite nice.

Because I am so tired. Of everything. But mostly of trying to remember.

My husband drifts into my head again, though I can't fully picture his face. Never mind. I'm sure someone will call him. I'm sure that when I wake up, he will be here.

85.

Josh

December 2036

We've gone easy on the Christmas decorations this year, not wanting to add to Rachel's confusion. There's a tree, lightly decked with baubles and a single string of silver bulbs. We keep the fire lit, because she likes that, even though she can no longer be left alone with naked flames, obviously. And that's about it. But I put *The Holiday* on for her yesterday, the volume turned low, and she seemed captivated. From time to time, when I looked up, her eyes were dancing, as if she was remembering how it feels to be enchanted.

The night before Christmas Eve, Emma comes into the kitchen with her partner, Kai. He's a barristers' clerk – though not from Emma's chambers – and is just about the most straightforward and uncomplicated guy I have ever met. They've been dating a couple of years now, and I am gutted that Rachel will never truly get to know him. Because all she ever wanted was for Emma to be happy.

I've been cooking all day, attempting to recreate Rachel's favourite kind of everything for the festive period. It's doubtful she'll eat much, but I can't not try. So the kitchen right now is a fug of simmering bread sauce, cranberries stewing in sugar, cheese straws fresh from the oven.

'Taste these,' I say to Emma and Kai, holding out a plate of mince pies.

Emma peers at them, wrinkles her nose. 'Are they—'

'Chocolate and chili. They're Rupert What's-his-name's.' (A sort of Heston disciple, who releases strange recipes each December for things like reindeer milk ice cream and quinoa Christmas puddings.)

Emma and Kai both laugh and back away slightly, as though the whole point of Christmas isn't to stuff your face with food that has a fifty-fifty chance of making you retch.

Then Emma says, 'Josh, Kai and I have something to tell you.'

I suspected a few weeks ago, once Emma started turning down wine at dinner and sleeping in past five a.m. But I said nothing, not wanting to pre-empt the announcement I felt sure was coming.

Now, I see the wild joy on her face – she is usually so self-contained, so composed – and feel happiness blaze through me like a firework. Her blue eyes are burning with excitement, cheeks plump with a smile she can't hold back. 'We're expecting twins.'

We rarely hug, Emma and I. She's just not really tactile like that. But today she makes an exception. 'Congratulations, both of you,' I say, as we put our arms around each other. Over her shoulder, I nod at Kai. Eyes sparkling, he nods right back. 'When are you due?'

'Six months,' she says, the timbre of her voice dipping slightly. Because we both know what that means. That maybe six months will be too late.

I try never to let my mind go there. Even during the awfulness of last summer, when Giles passed away after his cancer recurred, I refused to picture it. What Rachel's death will look like. How it will feel to be forced to absorb the fact of it. I resist – as I have always done – imagining her funeral, or saying goodbye, or the shape our lives will take without her.

It was weird, when Giles died. Even at his funeral, I couldn't cry. I think a big part of me simply couldn't accept he was gone. Maybe I had convinced myself, deep down, that somehow he might have found a way to live forever, too. That in five hundred years' time, he would still be by my side.

When Rachel first became ill, I was afraid I would eventually forget the person she used to be. But I see glimmers of the old her all the time. The way her eyes follow Emma around the room, bright and hopeful, as they have her whole life. The kind of food she loves to eat – Tunnock's Teacakes still a winner, as is pasta with obscene amounts of cheese. How she tries to scan even the direst situations for humour. That she cares if she makes a mess, because someone else will be cleaning it up. That, when she's trying to think, her eyes always stray to the nearest window – though what's going through her head now is anyone's guess. And that when Polly and Lo come over, or Ingrid dials in, her mood never fails to lift, and she always ends up laughing.

Tonight, though, once I'm back home, I find myself swamped with sadness. Rachel loves her daughter so deeply, and it kills me that she will never get to share in Emma's excitement about the babies. Her illness has robbed Rachel of the only thing she would ever have wanted – to hold and love and dote upon her grandchildren with her whole heart. So perhaps it is best that this all happened so quickly, before she knew anything about the part which would have broken her the most.

She is still here though, and still herself. She is simply an alternative version. And maybe that's true of us, too. We are changing every day, just as Rachel is. Doing life differently, trying our best to see the world through her eyes. None of us is the person we were before all this happened.

I no longer correct Rachel's mistakes, unless there's an imminent risk to life, obviously. I feel bad, now, for all the times I did. How much it must have confused her.

So when she asks me, occasionally, if we're still going to Aruba, I always say yes. And it's not wholly a lie. I tell her I'm looking forward to the moment we can finally watch that Caribbean sunset together, her hand in mine, sand between our toes.

86.

Rachel

December 2036/August 2003

I dream I am back at Josh's flat, thirty-three years ago. The home we used to share. The air throbs with electricity, the sky haemorrhaging rain.

Two days have passed since my argument with Lawrence. We've been seeing each other for seven months or so, and I am already filled with doubt.

'Sorry,' Josh says, reaching for a bottle of brandy, once I've finished telling him about it. 'Kind of feels like it's my fault.'

I know – of course I know – that it is chaotic and unfair, showing up at his flat unannounced, to complain about the row I've had with my new boyfriend. But that is not the true reason I came here tonight.

I want to tell him I made a mistake. That what I have with Lawrence can never come close to what we had. I want to know if there's a chance he will take me back.

But when he asks why I am here, the words feel too big for my throat, the room, this night. So I just end up saying weakly, 'I wanted a friend.'

With the curtains shut, by the scant light of a single lamp, we drink. Josh doesn't seem to mind that I've turned up like this, or maybe he's just humouring me. Selfishly, I'm not too sure I even care, because sitting in this living room, sharing brandy with our knees touching, is exactly what I need tonight.

After an hour or so, I say, 'Thank you for the clothes.'

I have changed into a pair of Josh's joggers and an old T-shirt, and we have spread out my wet stuff to dry in the kitchen, across various chairs and surfaces.

'That's all right,' he says, dark eyes skating over me. 'You always did rock that Teenage Fanclub T-shirt.'

I sip my drink. How can it be accidental that he has lent me this one – the same T-shirt he was wearing on the day I walked out?

But I don't comment on this. Instead, I say, 'By the way. I do know I shouldn't be here.'

He just lets out a soft laugh.

'What?' I say nervously.

He rubs the back of his neck, then draws a hand through his dark hair. 'Nothing. Not you, honestly. Just a touch of déjà vu. Don't worry about it.'

As I am trying to work out what he means, he says, 'The other night. I came back here with someone, but then she told me she'd been engaged less than a week.'

I unscrew the bottle cap and lean over to top him up. 'Oh, my God. What did you do?'

'Er, just watched her have an existential crisis then leave.'

I frown down at my glass. 'It's weird hearing about you sleeping with other people. I mean, I hate it, obviously.'

'Actually, you're specifically hearing about me *not* sleeping with other people. And you have just spent an hour talking to me about Lawrence.'

'I know. I'm a hypocrite. I do know that. But thinking about you having sex with other women just makes me jealous. I can't help it.'

'Yeah?' he murmurs, knocking back more brandy. 'It's all the other stuff that makes me jealous.'

'What other stuff?'

He lowers his glass, stares intently into it. The brandy has become smelted gold in the lamplight. 'I get jealous when you tell me about you and Lawrence hanging out with our friends, and going for dinner, and waking up together, and doing all the million little things I wish I was still doing with you, every single day.'

I swallow. The words burn on my tongue. *Let's try again, Josh.*

But then I think of Lawrence. The look on his face when I told him I needed a break. And all the reasons I left Josh come roaring back to me, and I know that, in reality, none of this – being here with him, talking and sharing eye contact and brandy together – means a single thing has changed between us.

So all I say is, 'I know. I'm sorry.'

He doesn't reply.

'But if it helps?' I smile faintly. 'I don't think our friends will ever be his friends.'

'No, they all think he's a twat,' he says, shooting me a wink and swigging again from his glass.

The hours pass, and we get drunker. Lawrence hasn't called. Outside, the night is a forest of falling rain.

'So, what is the sex like, with you and him?' Josh asks, shaking the last drops of brandy from the bottle. 'Just out of interest.'

'Nope. Not going there.'

'Don't be shy. You've told me everything else. Plus, we're so drunk. I won't remember in the morning.'

I skin my throat with more booze. 'The sex is fine, thanks.'

'Come on, Rach. I can take it.' He shrugs, wildly. 'We are where we are, right?'

'Okay. Well, sometimes it feels like we're not in sync. Emotionally, not—'

'—rhythmically. Right.'

To Josh's credit, he doesn't immediately begin shit-talking Lawrence, even though I've handed him the opportunity on a plate.

'Sometimes, it feels like we're just . . . shagging. You know? I mean, don't get me wrong. That can be okay.'

'Like when you just want—'

'—a shag. Exactly. But Lawrence only really has . . . that one gear. If you know what I mean.' I glance up, and as Josh's eyes latch to mine I feel something bright streak through me. A lightning bolt in my bloodstream.

'I do, actually,' he says.

'Please don't look at me like that.'

Smiling softly, he runs a hand along his jaw, lamplight pooling against his bare arms. 'Okay. But just so you know? I have . . . *so* many gears.'

Outside, icy ribbons of rain hound the windows.

'Josh, if we—'

'One time only. No strings. We're drunk.'

I nod and bite my lip. All logic and principles begin to warp and buckle in the heat of his gaze. 'And we are still married.'

'Right. I mean, does it even technically count?'

'Plus, we're on a break. Lawrence and me.'

'And he does only have one gear.'

At last he leans over and kisses me, and *God*, the familiar and delicious pressure of it, the heat of his palm on the back of my neck, the dizzying clasp of his mouth on mine. His tongue tastes sweet and ripe from the brandy. Our breath quickens, and I move in closer, not wanting an atom of space to remain between us.

His hand strays to my still-damp hair, then inside the T-shirt he has lent me, fingers teasing my rapidly warming skin. I run a hand over his muscles, feel them shudder and flex with my touch. And it is like falling into a thunderstorm, all electricity and shifting cells and crackling heat.

When eventually he moves to tease away my joggers, I inhale sharply, hesitate. 'Wait. We should keep our clothes on.'

In my head, I am reasoning – albeit with drunk-person logic – that if we're not naked it makes what we are doing less reprehensible, somehow. But I also can't deny I like the idea of it: fucking each other fast, clothes and underwear lowered just enough, like we might get caught at any moment.

'So, you do just want a shag?' Josh breathes, but his eyes are animated, as though he's down with that if I am.

'No.' I arch up into his kiss again. 'It's never just a shag with you.'

Afterwards, I am first to speak, though my mouth is brittle from the brandy, my words sticking together in slurs. We are still on the sofa, and he is lying on his back, eyes clamped shut, one hand resting on his forehead.

'I think . . . I should sleep in here,' I say.

It's difficult to know why, exactly. Maybe it's just instinct telling me that to wake up in Josh's arms tomorrow, without half a bottle of brandy inside me, would be too hard – and that the first thing we would want to do is the one thing we must never do again.

He nods and reaches clumsily down to rebutton his jeans, buckle his belt. 'Fair enough. But you're having my bed. I'll sleep in here.'

I totter to the bedroom, where I collapse, fully dressed, on to his mattress. The flat falls quickly quiet. All I can hear is the crack of rain against the windows, a noise that sounds entirely like reproach.

And now, a full thirty-three years later, I sit bolt upright in my bed.
    I know the truth of it instantly.
    Emma is not Lawrence's daughter.
    She is Josh's.

87.

Rachel

December 2036

I dreamt about something important last night. So important, in fact, that my brain was churning with urgency when I woke. But by the time I'd remembered where I was, and the whole palaver of washing and going to the toilet and eating breakfast had been dealt with, the dream had vanished entirely from my mind.

But it was to do with Emma. I'm sure of it. Emma, and her father.

Why didn't I write it down? Do I have a notebook anywhere?

We are in the living room, where I always feel safe, and warm. Someone has lit the fire, though it wasn't me, because I'm not allowed.

There is a fir tree standing by the window. I quite like it. Lights are winking softly from its branches. But they are not winking the way eyes do, watchful and sinister. These lights are more like stars. Beyond the glass, the world creaks with cold, the ground and trees newly stiff with frost.

'I have something to tell you,' I say to Emma. Perhaps if I just start talking, what I need to remember will come to me.

'Okay,' she says, smiling brightly. 'What's that, Mum?'

I stare at her for a long time, trying to squeeze out the memory from wherever it has lodged, in some dark recess of my brain. The effort makes me frown. 'I can't remember.'

'Well, not to worry,' she says gently. 'We've actually got something we wanted to tell you too.'

I don't recognise the fair-haired man sitting next to her. He's not been here before, I don't think.

'Mum, Kai and I are expecting twins. You're going to be a grandmother.'

Expecting twins? I think. *What does that mean?*

'We can't wait for you to meet them.'

I straighten up a little. 'Who? Who's coming?'

There is a knock at the living-room door. It opens, and another man puts his head around it.

My heart leaps with certainty. Dark, calm, kind. It is him. I am sure of it.

They begin to spark in my brain – fresh little static shocks of memory.

That bottle of brandy. The clamour of the rain. A kiss we couldn't stop. Paint samples on a bedroom wall, those five funny flavours of vanilla.

'I wore your T-shirt,' I gasp, grabbing on to the final image before it wriggles forever from my mind. 'Teenage Fanclub.'

The dark-haired man goes very still.

'She's a bit confused. We've just told her,' Emma whispers.

The words, at last, shoot out of me. 'We had a baby.'

'Well, we're having twins, Mum,' Emma says, infuriatingly calm, almost talking over me. 'You're going to be a grandmother.'

Why does no one ever listen to me?

I feel frustration hammer against my ribcage like a fist. It's not impossible that I will scream.

'*No. We* had a baby,' I insist, looking right at the dark-haired man, making my words into bullets, because it is the only way. 'You and me.'

Emma's jaw inches open, and her blue eyes seem somehow to take over her entire face. Then she snaps her head around, blonde hair swinging fiercely with the motion, and stares at the man too.

Without saying anything, she gets to her feet, and together they leave the room.

It is quite unbelievable, really.

'How rude,' I say with a headshake to the other man, who remains where he is. 'Didn't they hear me?'

But he doesn't reply. He seems a bit shocked. And I must confess, it's quite an unusual and pleasant feeling, to for once not be the only one who is lost for words.

88.

Josh

December 2036

Emma turns to me as soon as we enter the kitchen. Kai has stayed behind in the living room with Rachel.

She shuts the door. 'What the hell was that?'

For a moment or two, I can't speak.

I wore your T-shirt. Teenage Fanclub.

We had a baby. You and me.

In the back of my mind, old memories begin to glint and then vanish, like cobwebs in frost. I wonder if this is how it feels to be Rachel. Seeing only the faintest, most fragile outline of things, and only then when the light is tipped just right.

'You and my mum never had a baby – did you?' Emma's eyes are insistent, unblinking. Momentarily, it is as though she has me in the dock.

'No. *No.* Of course not.'

Her shoulders sink a little. Relief, I assume. She is wearing her Christmas jumper today, a faded Scandi-knit, crimson with white snowflakes. She gets it out every year, because it was a present once from Rachel.

She bites her lip. 'God, but there was something—' Breaking off, she shakes her head.

'What is it? Tell me.'

She shrugs, slightly helplessly. 'She seemed so desperate for us to hear what she was saying. Her voice was so urgent. Usually she's just slightly vacant. You know?'

I do. I noticed it too. But Rachel's mind is such a jumble these days, it's getting harder and harder to reliably interpret her demeanour.

'There's no chance . . .?' Emma begins.

I wait.

'There was never any crossover? With you and my dad?'

My heart starts to beat abnormally hard. Is she asking what I think she's asking?

She spells it out, too impatient to wait for me to catch up. 'There's no possibility Lawrence isn't my dad?'

'*No*. Lawrence is one hundred per cent your father. Your mum is just confused.'

Emma looks abruptly exhausted. It's not hard to get why. She is pregnant, and caring virtually full-time for a mother who no longer really knows her. And now this. I want to put my arms around her, but with Emma I can never quite predict if she's going to stick an elbow into my stomach and tell me to get off.

'You promise?' she says.

'I promise. Me and your mum never—'

I break off.

Well, there was that one night. Obviously. The night I think Rachel is remembering. When she turned up in the rain after that stupid row with Lawrence and I lent her my Teenage Fanclub T-shirt. And yes, we drank a whole bottle of brandy, and I spent much of the next day with my head in the toilet. I'd pretty much blacked out after a certain point. But we'd woken up fully clothed, in separate beds. And Rachel was still really into Lawrence, albeit he'd been acting like a bell-end. It's never occurred to me that anything happened between us. I haven't given it a second thought. Not once. And neither has Rachel, as far as I'm aware. We never felt the need to discuss it, not in all the years since.

But, suddenly, it strikes me that the maths would tally.

My skin turns cold as snow.

No. Not a chance. For one thing, Emma is so much half Lawrence, it's scary.

'You never what?' Emma prompts.

'Nothing. There's no chance Lawrence isn't your dad.'

Somewhere in the room, a bulb is buzzing, incessant as an insect. I make a mental note to sort it, because it's the kind of noise that really winds Rachel up these days.

Emma lets out a breath. 'Okay. Okay.'

I smile. 'Little bit relieved there, are you?'

'Um, yeah. What with you being twenty-nine and everything.'

Fair point. I lean back against the worktop, try to recover from the past few minutes. My eyes land on Rachel's cookbooks, lined up along a shelf. Some of them are from when we were married. Delia, Nigella, *The Naked Chef.* The sight of them always stills my heart. Because, true to form, Rachel's house isn't groaning with stuff, the way my flat is, after nearly seventy years on the planet. She has kept the habit of a lifetime, only holding on to possessions that mean the most.

'Have you told your dad about the babies yet?'

Emma nods. 'Although, we're not actually speaking at the moment.'

'Why not?' Lawrence and Emma fall out pretty regularly – another reason I'm convinced they're related. Their rows are always fierce in a way that borders on primal, that would seem almost impossible without them sharing genetic code.

'Oh, you know. As soon as we told him, he started interrogating Kai. Coming up with all these outdated and inaccurate opinions about his job and why he doesn't have his own flat and all this other irritating, regressive, patriarchal bullshit.'

'He probably just feels bad that he's not around to give you a hug in person.'

Emma tilts her head. 'You know, you give people the benefit of the doubt more than anyone I've ever met.'

'Well. Lawrence isn't all bad.'

That said, I did overhear the end of a fairly painful phone conversation between him and Emma, a few weeks back.

'It's not about whether she recognises you or not,' she was saying.

Pause.

'You're my *parents*. You, and Mum.'

Pause.

'Yes, of course the money's incredibly helpful, but—'

Pause.

'Because I think Mum would like it. Yes. Yes. Okay. Fine. Let me know.'

She hung up, let out a long sigh. And the futility of the whole situation made me sad. *He has no idea what he's got*, was all I could think.

He sent flowers to Rachel last week, with a card that read, *Thinking of you at this terrible time x*. I found both items stuffed into the kitchen bin the following morning, sprinkled liberally with the leftovers from Emma's Indian takeaway.

I feel her scanning my face now. 'I bet you wish Mum took that pill too, don't you?'

I gaze out of the window for a couple of moments. The garden is steel-skied and powdered with frost, picturesque as a Christmas card.

'No,' I say truthfully. 'Because she never wanted to. Not in her heart. Anyway, if she had, and we'd stayed together, you might not exist. And you like existing, don't you?'

Emma smiles. 'Usually. Most days.'

I let out a short laugh. 'I try not to think about that stuff too much. Take it from me – there's no point wishing for things that can never come true.'

'Well, I do.' Her voice becomes a tremor. 'I wish . . . I could have Mum back for just one more day. So I could talk to her about the babies. So Kai could see what an incredible person she truly is. So I could tell her I love her, and know she's really heard it. So I could tell her . . . not to be afraid.'

Her words are a landslide. Momentarily, they crush me.

Eventually, I say, 'You can still say all that stuff to her. I think she does understand, deep down. I really think she does.'

I don't confess that I've started talking to Rachel while she's asleep. I tell her I never stopped loving her, that I'll join her in the next life. I always ask her to wait for me there. Because the only thing I want is to be with her again. To pick up right where we left off.

Emma wipes tears from her eyes. But they don't seem wholly like tears of sadness. They are tears of frustration as well. 'I'm not ready to lose her, Josh. This is all happening too soon. It's so fucking unfair.'

Rachel's carers have the radio on, tuned to one of those stations that's non-stop Christmas. The music switches to 'River' by Joni Mitchell.

I have to turn away, so Emma can't see my face.

89.

Josh

April 2037

One morning in spring, I am shocked to receive an email from Wilf. He sent it to my agent first, who forwarded it on with only a run of exclamation marks in the subject line, as he does whenever he's affronted, which is often.

When I open the email, I can see why – although I do have to laugh. Wilf tells me he's been sitting on his notes for *Graveyard Heart* for almost two decades, so he thought it was about time. The notes, which he's attached on a three-page document, are largely criticism and only partly constructive – not to mention entirely pointless, since he never even read a draft.

He informs me, too, that he'll be back in the UK later this summer, suggests we go for a drink.

If I agree, it will be the first time I have seen him in nearly thirty years. I wonder if, at last, he is feeling the need to reconnect with the only other person in the world who knows what it's like to be him – minus the Einstein-sized brain, obviously.

Wilf tells me he got married a few years ago, to Camila, a Spanish woman he met on the poker circuit. She's in her thirties, which I'm not too sure how I feel about, given that, like me, Wilf is – chronologically – pushing seventy. But I'm not going to judge. There have never been any rulebooks, after all, for what we did.

He's a dad now, to boys aged three and eighteen months. He attaches a photo of the four of them on a mountainside, the kids in toddler carrier packs, Camila and Wilf lifting hiking poles skyward. This amuses me, since Wilf always used to claim he was allergic to any form of exercise, that it brought him out in hives.

But I can't help thinking, now what? Is Wilf just planning on watching the three people he loves most in the world getting old and infirm and dying, exactly as I am having to do with Rachel?

In terms of my own future, practically speaking, I'm relatively fortunate. I've got savings, which I've been surviving on since Rachel got ill and I took a break from writing. But, looking ahead, I'm pretty sure retirement – as most people know it – won't be an option for me. At some point the DWP are bound to red-flag the pension I've deferred, since I'm pretty sure the government don't have the money to bankroll people with zero impulse control and indefinite lifespans.

I wonder if Wilf ever thought, over the years, that a pill like the one we took might have become mass-market by now. That we'd be living in a world where old age was nothing but a scar on the landscape of history.

It will be good to see him, I think. I have a feeling that by the time he makes it back here, I will be needing all the friends I can get.

90.

Josh

June 2037

We've been told Rachel is nearing the end.

She's been hospitalised with chest infections twice in the past six months, and is now confined to bed. Her breathing grates and chafes as she drifts in and out of consciousness. She murmurs things, from time to time. Lately, she has started asking where her rings are again, who has stolen them. I always promise her we'll look for them, which seems to reassure her, if only temporarily.

I stay constantly by her side, with a heavily pregnant Emma. The house buzzes with visitors – Polly and Darren, Lo and her girls, Emma's friends, and, once, even Oliver and his new partner, from whom I kept a judicious distance. Old neighbours and colleagues drop by too, and countless other people whose relationships to Rachel are unclear to me, until Emma fills me in. Ingrid and Sean fly back from LA and rent a flat down the road. Gifts proliferate everywhere – flowers and cookies, chocolates, scented candles.

I keep drifting off then jerking awake like a dog, terrified Rachel will pass away while I'm sleeping. Next to me, Emma does the same. Both of us are delirious now with exhaustion. Consequently, we have been talking absolute nonsense pretty much non-stop. Yesterday, Kai walked in to find me halfway through some kind of soliloquy about the Milton Keynes grid system as Emma snored next to me, dribbling on to the shoulder of my T-shirt.

'You know, it's funny,' Emma murmurs, at one point. 'That Mum asked you to look after me, if anything happened to her. I reckon it'll be the other way around.'

I'd love to prove Emma wrong. But the truth is, I've no idea how I'll fare after Rachel is gone. I have only a handful of memories from my life before she was in it.

Still. No need to offload my entirely avoidable problems on to someone heavily pregnant with twins.

'I think you're going to have your hands full enough,' I say, plucking a shard of chocolate from the foil between us. Together, we have been destroying a leftover Easter egg that started out almost as big as my head. Of this, I feel sure Rachel would approve.

Next to us, Rachel starts to stir. She's become pretty restless over the past few days. The palliative team have told us this is probably because her organs are beginning to fail.

I hate hearing them say stuff like that. But Emma was firm about wanting the facts. Straight up, never sugar-coated. I guess she's advocated in enough cases of stabbings and stranglings and hammer-wielding lunatics to be immune, on some level, to bodies being reduced to blood, flesh, bones.

My eyes stray to the collection of Rachel's artwork on the wall. The embankment, splashed with watercolour. Geese on a lake in winter. And the front aspect of our old flat, the place I still call home. Bright blue front door, roses scaling the brickwork. The Victorian sash window she used to love looking out of.

I turn my gaze to Rachel again. Her greying hair is a cloud on the pillow, the lines on her face like the staves of a song. I hope her mind is stirring only with beautiful music, memories of a life well-lived.

But, as I'm looking down at her, Rachel begins trying – with much effort, and quite out of nowhere – to speak. To say my name, and then her daughter's.

Emma straightens up, swings a hand on to my arm, grips hard.

Rachel blinks twice. Her eyes swim, their burnt-sugar brown unchanged since the day we met.

She draws a long breath and swallows, moistens her lips. Then: 'Josh.'

Impossibly, her voice is clear as an alpine stream.

91.

Rachel

June 2037

Like a rescue flare into a darkened sky, my mind has roared to life.

Synapses stir. Pathways swell and expand, cells remember.

Yes, I think. *I have a daughter, and a loving family, and two grandchildren on the way.*

I feel a hand grip mine. And it is a hand I know well, by its gentle weight, the geography of its palm. The cool kiss of a watch strap. I feel with my thumb for the writer's bump, and find it straight away: that soft knot, right middle finger.

And a soulmate, I think, a smile surfacing on my lips. *I have a soulmate, too.*

'Josh,' I say. And then, because I can't quite believe I have managed to form a word, I repeat it, louder this time. 'Josh.'

All my senses are suddenly primed. Summer tumbles through the propped-open window, a hot, bright light. The scent of freshly chopped grass and roses in bloom, laundry billowing on the breeze.

How long have I been asleep?

'I need to talk to you both.' My throat creaks a little before my voice locates its groove. 'I've been thinking about something that happened, thirty-three years ago.'

Emma gasps and covers her mouth, tears clinging to the edges of her eyes.

I grab her pale, slim hand and try to squeeze it, though I barely have the strength. 'Don't cry, darling.'

She just shakes her head, seemingly unable to reply.

'Rachel,' Josh says softly. 'How are you feeling?'

'I'm tired,' I say, with a laugh that rattles. 'So very tired.'

It's lovely to see him again. I admit, I sometimes envied his youth, over the years. His sharp jaw and firm limbs, the little belts of muscle. Skin still taut, hair resolutely dark. How his bones and blood remained healthy, his mind new. The way sunlight on his face always made him look younger and not older.

Yes, I have wanted all that. If only for a snatched moment, from time to time. Being young isn't better, necessarily. But sometimes, it is easier.

And here is Emma, too. My gorgeous, golden girl, who glows so hard she can warm any room.

I squeeze her hand more firmly now. 'Listen. I need you to hear this. Both of you.' I clear my throat, attempt to still the jump in my stomach. 'There was a night that year, in August, when Josh and I . . . Do you remember, Josh?'

As Josh brings his gaze to mine, I know he does. Not fully, perhaps, not yet – but I can see the faint heat of recollection is there, like a pulse.

'Lawrence and I had had a row. And I came to your flat, and we drank a whole bottle of brandy. The one you'd bought your mum, for her birthday.'

Realisation begins to inch across his face. 'Yeah. That's right. Messy night.'

'Very messy night. I threw up in your kitchen sink the next day. Twice.'

He laughs softly. 'I'd forgotten about that. Had to . . . never mind.'

'Anyway, we woke up fully clothed in different beds, so we ended up deciding . . . that nothing had happened.'

Josh shifts in his chair. He glances at Emma, then back at me.

'But something did happen.'

Neither of them speaks.

Emma's face has become rigid, almost translucent. She is sitting up very straight, her stomach huge and boulder-like in her lap.

'I think you should get a DNA test.'

'Oh, my God,' Josh breathes. His knuckles blanch as he grips the seat of his chair, veins leaping on the tops of his hands.

'That night came back to me, in a kind of dream.' I meet his gaze, draw it close. 'We did sleep together. You might not remember, but I do.'

Emma puts one hand to her stomach and the other to her mouth.

'No, Rachel. You wouldn't have wanted that.' Josh's voice is darting everywhere, like a leaf on a breeze. 'You and Lawrence—'

'I know. But I need you to take a test. Just . . . promise me you'll take a test.'

The air shimmers with shock. Wordlessly, Josh and Emma share a look.

I have more to say, and apologise for. But my eyes seem to want to close.

'I love you,' I whisper to Josh.

'I love you too.' His voice shakes and breaks, sinking into me in slivers.

And then I whisper the other thing I have to tell him, at which he covers his face with one hand, and begins to cry.

'And Emma,' I say. Her name is warm water to the muscle of my heart. She has blown my mind every day since she was born. 'I love you so much. Enjoy it all, darling. You're going to be an incredible mum. I'm just so sorry this didn't come to me sooner.'

I take in the sight of them for a final time, then close my eyes.

92.

Josh

June 2037

A few seconds after Rachel slips back into unconsciousness, Emma stands up and leaves the room.

I watch Rachel for a moment to check she's still breathing, then wipe my eyes and go to find Emma. On the landing, I pass Rachel's nurse. She smiles peacefully at me, as if life as we all know it hasn't just been drop-kicked into outer space.

Halfway down the stairs, I hear the back door close. Emma clearly needs time, and to be honest so do I.

I try to busy myself in the kitchen for a while. Briefly I wonder if, together, we hallucinated the whole thing. Conjured it up between us, a mirage made from pure exhaustion.

Eventually, Emma comes back inside.

A streak of normality follows her in through the open door. Breeze-tossed linen, birds gossiping, sky saturated with sunshine. No hint of shadows, or dark pasts.

She crosses the kitchen, lowers herself into a chair.

I wait for her to speak, because I owe her that much.

'You said there was no chance,' she says eventually.

I feel her eyes on me, the endless blue burn of them. 'I honestly didn't think there was.'

'How drunk were you?'

'Quite. I mean, very.'

'Blackout?'

I feel like a teenager she's cross-examining, as though I'm moments from being slapped with an ASBO. 'Probably. I have no memories past a certain point.'

'But Mum does, apparently.' She shakes her head, looks away from me.

'I'm sorry.' It's a weird thought: that I let her down before she was even born. The consequences of being too pissed to remember coming back to bite us all, more than three decades down the line. 'I know this must be a shock.'

'What just happened up there?' she says, confusion spilling everywhere. 'Mum was almost herself again. I haven't seen her like that in *years*.' A sob chokes out of her, and she smothers it, too late, with a hand.

Worry stirs in my stomach, concern for the babies. Surely they recommend sidestepping emotional landmines when you're heavily pregnant? And don't twins often show up early?

'Look . . .' I attempt to say something reassuring. 'Maybe how your mum was just now means she's turning a corner.'

Hope, always. An unburst bud in my chest.

Emma shakes her head. 'That's impossible.'

'We don't know. Let me talk to the nurse, and maybe we can—'

'Josh. Wait.'

The room, temporarily, feels as though it is floating. Suspended in the hinterland between two opposing versions of our reality.

'You and my dad did look awfully alike,' she says. 'Back in the day. Mum said people used to joke she'd replaced you with a lookalike. No offence.'

I decide, just for once, to let this outrageous slander slide. 'But you're very similar to Lawrence, Emma. In lots of ways.'

'No, that's what I'm saying. Maybe I don't look like Lawrence. Maybe I look like you.'

'I meant, personality-wise.'

She shrugs. 'Nature or nurture, though?'

'Nature,' I say firmly.

'You and Mum both have brown eyes,' she says slowly. 'And I have blue.'

Like most normal people, I know next to nothing about inherited eye colour. Though, for some inexplicable reason, I do seem to remember that Lawrence's eyes are green. Is that closer to blue, genetically? I have no idea.

'You honestly can't remember anything about that night?'

'Bits and pieces. Not much. And nothing to do with me and your mum . . .'

'Getting it on?'

I lean back against the worktop, almost feeling a blush coming on. 'Sure. If that's what the kids are calling it these days.'

A smile creeps over her face. 'Look at you getting bashful.'

'Must we.'

'Did you really drink a whole bottle of brandy?'

'I think so. The hangover's the only part I do remember.'

'Half a bottle of brandy would kill me.'

'It almost killed me.'

'We should take that test.'

'Emma—'

'I'm serious, Josh. I need to know. Don't you?'

I do, of course. But at the same time, I cannot even begin to compute that this brilliant and shining woman could possibly be my daughter.

Then again, we've all been happy to assume she's Lawrence's. Which is equally ludicrous, if you ask me.

'Will you go out and get one? Please?'

'Okay. I will. But there's something I need to do first.'

I tell her what I've been thinking about for a few days now.

She listens carefully, then nods. 'Yes. Thank you. I think that would be a really lovely thing to do.'

93.

Rachel

June 2037

I open my eyes. And at last: there they are.

My wedding and engagement rings, in a little glass dish on my nightstand.

I reach out and pick them up, nearly dropping them as I do so, because I am really quite useless at holding things now.

Eventually, with shaking hands, I manage to slide them on to my ring finger. They are a little loose, which is odd. I can't remember taking them off. But that's hardly surprising. It's a struggle to recall very much at all any more.

And then, quite out of nowhere, I feel a kind of dreamy peace wash over me. Calm and warm, like spreading out a picnic blanket on a summer's day.

I turn to my nightstand again, open the drawer, and lift out the love letter I have kept for . . . Well. Let's just say, it's been a very long time.

I struggle to read now. But that doesn't matter. Because I can recite this letter by heart. I just like the feeling of holding the paper in my hand, exactly as Josh would have done, all those years ago.

Hey, Rachel,

It was amazing to meet you, the other week. I'd really love to see you again. I sort of can't stop thinking about you . . . ! Hope that's not too much. But I couldn't not tell you.

I feel like this could be something pretty epic.
Here's my address, and number.

Yours hopefully,
J xx

Shakily, I fold the letter up again, then slide it back inside the envelope with my university address on the front, and the nineteen-pence stamp.

I glance at the clock on the wall. It's nearly five p.m. That means it won't be long until Josh gets home from teaching. The last thing he did before leaving the house was lift my hand and kiss my knuckle, just as he did at the end of his speech on our wedding day. I remember that so clearly.

He told me he'd be back soon.

There is a vase of roses on the windowsill. He cuts them for me every summer, from the bushes he tends in our garden.

Outside, the sunlight is starting to soften. But the sky remains a tranquil, effortless blue. I can hear birds chattering, a distant dog bark, children playing. The tempting scent of a barbecue. It must be weeks since we had one. Perhaps I'll ask Josh if he fancies that, this weekend.

My mind is beginning to slide now, slipping down a slope leading only to sleep.

I hope he's had a good day, I think, as I feel myself go. We'll cook something nice tonight, when he gets in. Have a glass of wine and watch the sun set together, his hand in mine.

94.

Josh

June 2037

Before I left the house just now, I set Rachel's rings into a little glass dish on her nightstand while she slept. I asked Emma's permission to do so, of course. She said yes without hesitation, fetched the rings for me from Rachel's jewellery box.

I hoped they would be the first thing she saw, the next time she opened her eyes.

I took her left hand and kissed it softly, on the knuckle of her ring finger, exactly as I did on our wedding day.

'Bye, Rach,' I whispered. 'I'll be back soon.'

They sell DNA analysis kits in supermarkets these days. It'll take a week or so for the results to come through, once we've sent off the samples. But they sit right alongside the pregnancy tests.

I grab one, and then another for luck. My heart strobes painfully, in time with the supermarket strip-lighting.

But when I get back to Rachel's house, Emma is sitting on the front step.

She is crying, her face contorted.

No.

No, no, no, no, no.

'She's gone.' Her voice is shattered by sobs. 'Ten minutes ago. She's gone. I'm so sorry, Josh.'

Dropping the tests, I sink to my knees, right where I am in the middle of the drive.

I put my head in my hands, let everything go.

95.

Josh

June 2037

Terminal lucidity, the doctor said. It's a thing, apparently. As dementia patients near the end, they can occasionally sit up and begin to converse clearly. Almost return to their old selves.

This lucidity can last from a couple of hours to several days. But, even after decades of research, the medical profession is no closer to figuring out exactly what brings it on.

I wish I'd known it was even a possibility. That way, I could have set my shock aside, and just enjoyed Rachel coming back to us, one last time. Exactly as she always was.

It's been six days since she died. Perhaps unsurprisingly, Emma's waters broke early the next morning. She's still in hospital now.

It is almost impossible, I have discovered, to digest grief and joy at the same time. Swallowed together, they are too big, too hot, too raw. So I just do laps of my flat, the park, the river, trying to sweat the feelings out of me.

It never works. They don't go anywhere. The heartburn rages on.

I can't stop replaying the last thing Rachel whispered to me, on the day she died. 'I told you once that I didn't want to be ninety and still thinking about you, Josh. But it wasn't true. You were my favourite thing to think about. Always.'

Emma has given birth to a girl and a boy. The first time I called, she told me they had named the girl Florence Rachel Carmichael.

'Beautiful. And the boy?' I asked.
'Ezra Josh Carmichael.'
'Oh, Emma.'
'I think Mum would have approved, don't you?'
As it happens, I do.

We took the DNA test just hours after Rachel passed away. In that moment, everything felt surreal, the world jumbled up. An optical illusion, making origami of our brains.

When I expressed this to Emma, she just said, 'Shut up and swab your damn mouth, will you?'

At this, despite everything, I had to laugh.

She calls the day after she and the twins are out of hospital. 'I've got the email. I haven't opened it yet.'

'There's no rush. Take your time.' I don't mean a word of this, of course.

'When have you ever known me to take my time?'
Fair point. 'Shall I come over?'
I hear her smile down the line. 'Did you think we were going to do this over the phone?'

And so it is that, in the presence of Emma and her six-day-old twins, I discover I am a father and a grandfather at exactly the same time.

Emma cries straight away, assures me with a smile it isn't personal. I laugh through my own tears, then put out my arms. She creeps between them, sets her head on my shoulder. She smells of grief and happiness, a life forever changed.

'I guess two browns can make a blue,' she says.

'I guess so,' I say with a smile. 'Who knew?'

The babies squirm slightly on the table, in seats designed to bounce. They seem entirely unfazed by our bombshell, perhaps even a little bored.

I press a kiss into her hair. 'How do you reckon Lawrence will take it?'

'Badly, I should think.'

'He'll still love you no matter what, you know.' Because how could he not?

She draws back, gazes up at me. She looks tired, but happy too. 'You have grandchildren,' she whispers.

Emma and Kai have decided to live at Rachel's for a month or so, while they recover and get settled with the twins. I offer to stay for a few days, to help out. Emma lets me have Rachel's room.

Nobody has been in it since the day she died.

Opening the door, I step inside.

I go over to her bed, try to imagine lying down in the space she has left. Attempting sleep, then waking tomorrow, remembering she is gone, the pain like swallowing broken glass.

Dusk and silence have flooded the room now. Downstairs, even the babies are taking a breather from bawling in stereo.

Through the gloom, I let my gaze explore, lingering on every detail. The final bunch of flowers I brought her, blush-pink roses from our old garden, wilting now on the windowsill, their heads bowed in grief. All of my books, lined up on a shelf. The painting she did of me and Emma, hand in hand on an ice rink one Christmas.

Rachel must have found the rings where I'd left them, because she was wearing them when she died. The thought both burns and comforts me.

I feel around in my pocket, then take out my own wedding ring. I hold it in my outstretched palm, just for a second, then slip it on to my finger for the first time in twenty-five years.

Next to the ring dish is my favourite photo of the two of us, in each other's arms on the dance floor at Polly's son's wedding. My daughter must have taken it, though I didn't know it at the time. My *daughter*.

In the photo, the air is tinted gold by a million lights. Rachel is smiling, maybe in response to something I have said. I wish I could remember what.

But the thing that strikes me most is that we don't look odd, or incongruous, or in any way remarkable.

We look just right.

Acknowledgements

I would like to say a huge thank you to Rebecca Ritchie at A M Heath, forever my champion and confidante, for all your guidance and support, and wise words when they're needed most. To Euan Thorneycroft, for your feedback and sound advice when I first pitched the idea for this book (and for not telling me it was far too bonkers to ever make it into print). To Phoebe Morgan, Tallulah Lyons and Jake Carr at Hodder, for your invaluable input, insight and ideas, which helped to shape this novel into the reading experience I always wanted it to be. To Kit Nevile, for your passion, enthusiasm and sage editorial suggestions – thank you for 'getting' this story from the start, and for truly understanding what lay at its heart. To Linda McQueen, for diligent and astute copyediting, and Chere Tricot for eagle-eyed proofreading. I owe immense gratitude too, as always, to the whole wider team at Hodder, for your care and hard work. And to my husband Mark, for your unwavering faith, and for everything else.

Some novels are hard to write – even if the resulting read might seem effortless. *Still Falling For You* was not one of these; in fact, the whole experience felt closer to pure joy, from start to finish. I wrote the first draft in something of a creative fever, during March three years ago over a shockingly short number of days, unable to leave my keyboard for twelve hours at a time, often longer. Rachel and Josh's love story had taken hold of me, and was refusing, quite wonderfully, to let go. For that reason, this book has, and will always have, my heart. I hope that when you reach the final page, you feel the same. Thank you, as always, for reading.

**Breathtaking love stories
by bestselling author Holly Miller**

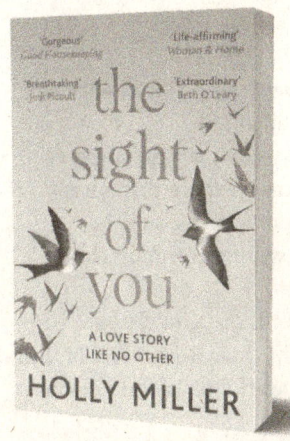

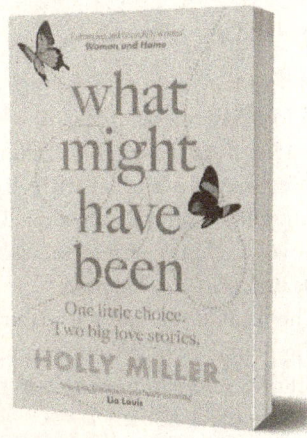

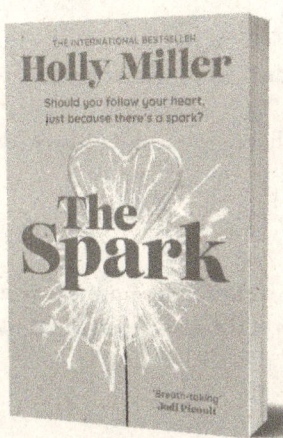

Discover your next obsession today!

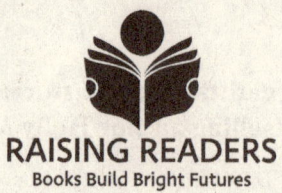

RAISING READERS
Books Build Bright Futures

Dear Reader,

We'd love your attention for one more page to tell you about the crisis in children's reading, and what we can all do.

Studies have shown that reading for fun is the **single biggest predictor of a child's future life chances** – more than family circumstance, parents' educational background or income. It improves academic results, mental health, wealth, communication skills, ambition and happiness.[1]

The number of children reading for fun is in rapid decline. Young people have a lot of competition for their time. In 2024, 1 in 10 children and young people in the UK aged 5 to 18 did not own a single book at home.[2]

Hachette works extensively with schools, libraries and literacy charities, but here are some ways we can all raise more readers:

- Reading to children for just 10 minutes a day makes a difference
- Don't give up if children aren't regular readers – there will be books for them!
- Visit bookshops and libraries to get recommendations
- Encourage them to listen to audiobooks
- Support school libraries
- Give books as gifts

There's a lot more information about how to encourage children to read on our website: **www.RaisingReaders.co.uk**

Thank you for reading.

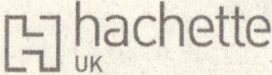

---

[1] OECD, '21st-Century Readers: Developing Literacy Skills in a Digital World', 2021, https://www.oecd.org/en/publications/21st-century-readers_a83d84cb-en.html

[2] National Literacy Trust, 'Book Ownership in 2024', November 2024, https://literacytrust.org.uk/research-services/research-reports/book-ownership-in-2024